DEVELOPMENT IN JEOPARDY

Clinical Responses to Infants and Families

Clinical Infant Reports
Series of the **ZERO TO THREE/** National Center for Clinical Infant Programs

Editorial Board

Stanley I. Greenspan, M.D., Chairman

Kathryn E. Barnard, R.N., Ph.D.
T. Berry Brazelton, M.D.
Anneliese Korner, Ph.D.
Jeree Pawl, Ph.D.
Sally Provence, M.D.
Jack Shonkoff, M.D.

Clinical Infant Reports is a series of book length publications of the **ZERO TO THREE**/National Center for Clinical Infant Programs designed for practitioners in the multidisciplinary field of infant health, mental health, and development. Each volume presents diagnostic and therapeutic issues and methods, as well as conceptual and research material.

DEVELOPMENT IN JEOPARDY

Clinical Responses to Infants and Families

Editors

Emily Fenichel, M.S.W.
Sally Provence, M.D.

International Universities Press, Inc.
Madison ● Connecticut

Library of Congress Cataloging-in-Publication Data

Development in jeopardy : clinical responses to infants and families / editors, Emily Fenichel, Sally Provence.
    p. cm. — (Clinical infant reports series of the Zero to Three/National Center for Clinical Infant Programs)
    Includes bibliographical references and index.
    ISBN 0-8236-1227-9
    1. Infant psychiatry—Case studies. 2. Child psychiatry—Case studies. 3. Infants—Mental health services—Case studies. 4. Toddlers—Mental health services—Case studies. 5. Child development deviations—Prevention—Case studies. 6. Maternal and infant welfare—Case studies. I. Fenichel, Emily Schrag. II. Provence, Sally, 1916–   . III. Series: Clinical infant reports.
    [DNLM: 1. Child Psychology—case studies. 2. Child Development—
case studies. 3. Parents—psychology. 4. Child Psychiatry—case studies. WS 350 D4843 1993]
    RJ502.5.D48 1993
    362.2′0425—dc20
    DNLM/DLC
for Library of Congress   93-2032
                                           CIP

International Universities Press and IUP (& design) ® are registered trademarks of International Universities Press, Inc.
Manufactured in the United States of America

Dedication

Sally Provence, a founding member of the National Center for Clinical Infant Programs, the first editor of its bulletin, *Zero to Three,* president of **ZERO TO THREE/** National Center for Clinical Infant Programs from 1985 to 1988, and editor of *Infants and Parents: Clinical Case Reports* (Clinical Infant Reports Number Two), died in February, 1993. She had trained directly, or guided and inspired, generations of individuals who are now working with young children and their families. During her years of illness, Sally Provence continued to guide the editing of the case reports that are included in this volume, and to conceptualize and articulate her ideas of what constitutes a "clinical response" to infants and parents.

Sally Provence's compassion, wisdom, and deep respect for the power and complexity of human development have helped to inspire what is best in all the work reported here. More than anyone else, she embodied in her own "clinical responses," as well as in her research and writings, what have become guiding principles for clinical work with, and enlightened policies toward, infants, young children, and their families. Those of us who learned from her directly feel privileged as we try to share her vision with new generations of children, families, and those who care for them.

Stanley I. Greenspan, M.D.
Chairman
Editorial Board, *Clinical Infant Reports*

ZERO TO THREE/National Center for Clinical Infant Programs is the only national nonprofit organization dedicated solely to improving the chances for healthy physical, cognitive and social development of infants, toddlers, and their families.

Established in 1977, **ZERO TO THREE** is committed to:

○ exercising leadership in developing and communicating a national vision of the importance of the first three years of life and of the importance of early intervention and prevention to healthy growth and development;

○ developing a broader understanding of how services for infants and toddlers and their families are best provided; and

○ promoting training in keeping with that understanding.

Contents

Contributors

Jean Adnopoz, M.P.H., Associate Clinical Professor, Child Study Center, Yale University, New Haven, Connecticut.

Peter Blos, Jr., M.D., Training Analyst and Adult and Child Supervising Analyst, Michigan Psychoanalytic Institute; Lecturer, Department of Psychiatry, University of Michigan, Ann Arbor, Michigan.

Elsa J. Blum, Ph.D., Adjunct Assistant Professor of Psychology and Psychiatry, The New York Hospital–Cornell Medical Center, Westchester Division, White Plains, New York; private practice, Roslyn, New York.

T. Berry Brazelton, M.D., Clinical Professor of Pediatrics, Emeritus, Harvard Medical School, Boston, Massachusetts.

Douglas Davies, Ph.D., M.S.W., Social Work Specialist and Lecturer, Infancy and Early Childhood Program, Department of Psychiatry, University of Michigan Medical Center; Adjunct Assistant Professor, School of Social Work, University of Michigan, Ann Arbor, Michigan.

Emily Fenichel, M.S.W., Associate Director, **ZERO TO THREE**/National Center for Clinical Infant Programs, Arlington, Virginia.

Barbara Fields, M.A., M.S.W., Private practice, New Rochelle, New York and New York City.

Margie Morrison, LCSW, Private practice, Chicago, Illinois; Department of Psychiatry, The University of Chicago.

Jeree H. Pawl, Ph.D., Clinical Professor, Director, Infant–Parent Program, San Francisco General Hospital, University of California at San Francisco.

Sally Provence, M.D., Professor Emerita, Yale University Child Study Center, New Haven, Connecticut.

Chaya H. Roth, Ph.D., Associate Professor of Clinical Psychiatry, University of Chicago Medical Center; Founder and Senior Consultant, Parent–Infant Development Service, Department of Psychiatry, University of Chicago Medical Center.

Helen Scharfman, M.S.W., Program Director, Parent/Child Program, Lexington Center for Mental Health Services, Inc., Jackson Heights, New York.

Jack P. Shonkoff, M.D., Professor of Pediatrics, Chief, Division of Developmental and Behavioral Pediatrics, University of Massachusetts Medical School, Worcester, Massachusetts.

Albert J. Solnit, M.D., Sterling Professor Emeritus, Yale University Child Study Center, New Haven, Connecticut.

Fred R. Volkmar, M.D., Harris Associate Professor, Yale University Child Study Center, New Haven, Connecticut.

Preface

This volume is the sixth in the series of Clinical Infant Reports sponsored by **ZERO TO THREE**/National Center for Clinical Infant Programs. The series is designed especially for practitioners in the new and growing multidisciplinary field of infant health, mental health, and development.

Each volume in the series addresses an identified gap in the professional literature. Of special interest to the series are theoretical inquiries, empirical investigations, and in-depth case studies which relate to the challenges of clinical work with infants, young children, and their families.

Like Clinical Infant Reports Number 2, *Infants and Parents: Clinical Case Reports*, edited by Sally Provence, the current volume includes contributions from clinicians who represent a range of professional disciplines, work settings, and geographical areas—as do the readers of this series and of other publications of **ZERO TO THREE**/ National Center for Clinical Infant Programs. From this diversity emerges a common commitment, guiding both practice and research, to provide increasingly timely, responsive, and appropriate support to children and families in the earliest years of life.

Jeree H. Pawl, Ph.D., Clinical Professor, Director, Infant–Parent Program, San Francisco General Hospital, University of California at San Francisco.

Sally Provence, M.D., Professor Emerita, Yale University Child Study Center, New Haven, Connecticut.

Chaya H. Roth, Ph.D., Associate Professor of Clinical Psychiatry, University of Chicago Medical Center; Founder and Senior Consultant, Parent–Infant Development Service, Department of Psychiatry, University of Chicago Medical Center.

Helen Scharfman, M.S.W., Program Director, Parent/Child Program, Lexington Center for Mental Health Services, Inc., Jackson Heights, New York.

Jack P. Shonkoff, M.D., Professor of Pediatrics, Chief, Division of Developmental and Behavioral Pediatrics, University of Massachusetts Medical School, Worcester, Massachusetts.

Albert J. Solnit, M.D., Sterling Professor Emeritus, Yale University Child Study Center, New Haven, Connecticut.

Fred R. Volkmar, M.D., Harris Associate Professor, Yale University Child Study Center, New Haven, Connecticut.

Introduction

Each case report in this book begins with a child, or children, in the first three years of life, whose healthy development is in jeopardy. Each report then describes, in detail, the clinical response of one or more professionals to the infant, and to his family.

We hope that this volume will have meaning for at least two audiences. Practitioners whose daily work lies in providing services to individual infants and parents constitute our first intended audience. Students of infants, toddlers, and their families in a range of disciplines—senior researchers as well as undergraduates—comprise our second audience. Practitioners can find in these pages affirmation of the importance of their own work and that of others who use similar, and different, methods to provide effective, timely services. Practitioners, researchers, and students alike will find applications of theoretical understanding and reminders of the essential uniqueness of each infant and family. We have tried to use language that is specific while avoiding terminology that has meaning only to particular disciplines or adherents of particular theories.

The studies in this volume reinforce the view that the earliest years of life are a time of great vulnerability, but also an occasion for great hope. If an infant is living in an environment unfavorable for reasonably healthy growth

and development, his chances can be seriously jeopardized, and his well-being becomes more endangered the
longer inadequate caregiving or a noxious environment
persists. But when skilled help is available early to the
infant and family, positive change may be dramatic. Early
assistance, sometimes quite brief, can be truly curative.
The normal, forward thrust of development may be restored.

These case reports also reflect a view of parents as
individuals who themselves undergo a developmental process during their child's early years and beyond. The birth
of an infant and the experiences of early child rearing
evoke powerful responses in parents. Parents' responses
are influenced by their previous experiences of nurturing
and being cared for, by current realities in their life situation, by the support available to them from each other
and from other family members and friends, and by the
characteristics of the child himself, including any illness
or disability he might have. Raising an infant or toddler
provides an opportunity for adults to confront old issues
and to grow further. This process may be difficult, however, unless support is available.

There are many possible ways to support the development of young children and their parents, ranging from
federal income tax policies to health care to neighborly
assistance. What do we mean, then, when we use the
phrase "clinical responses to infants and parents"? As
readers of this volume will discover, such responses can be
made by professionals (and paraprofessionals) from many
different disciplines and from different theoretical orien-
tations within those disciplines. Responses can be offered
to infants and parents in hospitals, in homes, in social service agencies, and in courtrooms. Interventions may be
mild or intensive. Those working with the infant and family may use one or several approaches to assessment and
to treatment; they may work independently, as part of a

multidisciplinary team, or in a collaborative relationship with staff of several agencies. As various as these activities may appear, however, they have at least four important elements in common.

First, a clinical response rests on a conceptual framework for understanding developmental issues and problems in children and parents in the earliest years of life. It would be incorrect to assert that a single theory of infant development exists that would be agreed upon by all experts. Efforts to classify the developmental and psychopathological disorders of the earliest years are complicated by the fact that a particular clinical disorder may be caused by different conditions, and that similar conditions or factors can result in different clinical syndromes. Nevertheless a number of key principles and observations about early development have emerged as powerful integrators of information across fields of inquiry and as general guides, across disciplines, for practice with infants and families.

For example, observers of child development agree that multiple lines of development are not independent and separate, but rather interdependent and interactive, especially in the first three years of life. Consequently, parents, other caregivers, and therapists need to support growth within and across the areas of physical development, motility, cognition, speech, organization of experience, and emotional development.

Researchers and practitioners are also documenting with increasing specificity how the quality of the relationship between a baby and his caregivers affects the child's development in all areas. As a consequence, professional support and intervention is being focused more on the families of infants and toddlers. By strengthening and expanding the family's resources, energy, coping capacities, and nurturing skills, practitioners attempt to improve the relationship between parent and infant and, ultimately, the developmental outcomes for both parent and child.

"Temperament," "coping," "attachment," "transaction," "multiple risk," and "reciprocity" are additional concepts that are now part of the everyday vocabulary of practitioners who work with infants and families, even though these concepts seemed revolutionary only a decade or so ago. These principles and others are constantly being elaborated and refined.

The connection between key concepts and clinical practice should be evident, or at least traceable, in every encounter between professional and family, providing a rationale for the practitioner's words and actions. Then, if a verbal comment, a piece of concrete assistance, or the timing of an intervention seems helpful, one will have an idea of why this might be so. If an approach falls flat or behavior remains baffling, one can return to core concepts for fresh understanding, or, possibly, revision of one's hypotheses themselves.

Second, a clinical response must address the particular, unique needs of an individual child or family. There are many pressures to "standardize" assessment protocols, infant–toddler curricula, home visit discussion topics, and the like. But no matter how closely they reflect our best understanding about infants and families, assessment instruments, service program elements, and treatment procedures are tools, not ends in themselves. If they are not adapted appropriately, they may impede, rather than assist, the work.

Thus the clinician uses an assessment as a way to help answer a family's questions about particular aspects of a particular baby's development. The clinician seeks to understand not only what developmental milestones the child has achieved but also how he approaches new challenges, whether joyfully, reluctantly, or determinedly. The clinician also observes carefully what is going on between baby and caregiver as an assessment proceeds. In order to serve individual families appropriately, a clinically responsive program includes: accommodation in service delivery, whenever possible, to the particular circumstances at hand; cultural sensitivity; attention to families' expressed needs; and the flexibility to address issues that may only emerge over time. Since no single program or agency can meet all the needs of every infant or family who comes to its door, a clinical response may also involve helping a family negotiate to get what it needs from other sources.

Third, a clinical response involves awareness of, and reflection upon, the helping relationship itself. When a parent and another adult undertake to work together to foster a baby's development, a relationship begins that may be enormously powerful but also delicate. The feelings that are evoked in participant and service provider in any helping relationship tend to be intensified whenever the well-being of a baby is at issue. While mental health practitioners have given a great deal of thought to "the professional use of self" in therapeutic relationships, other disciplines concerned with young children and their families have at times focused more on the health, educational, or social services provided than on the relationships involved. This situation is changing. Increasing attention is being paid to the importance and quality of the parent–professional relationship itself as a vital influence in supporting the infant's development. Practitioners from a range of disciplines are reflecting upon their feelings and attitudes toward families, redefining their roles, and, perhaps most importantly, placing a higher value on their ability to create and sustain working relationships with multiply stressed families.

Finally, a clinical response takes place within a system of care that, ideally, supports the practitioner as well as the child and family. To undertake and persist in the difficult work of a reflective practice with infants and parents, professionals themselves need support. Just as we have learned to look at the infant in the context of the family, and the family in the context of its support network, so we must look at the practitioner in the context of the system of care in which she works. Virtually all clinicians begin with a basic desire to help. They learn to use both science and art to enable positive change to take place in infants and parents. To be effective over the long term, practitioners need not only the experience of matching increasing skills to demanding (but not overwhelming) clinical challenges, but also support from the institutions that offer services to young children and families and from the social policies that affect this population.

Training is important. The infant–family practitioner needs not only to command the skills of her particular discipline but also to be able to adapt these to specialized practice with babies and parents. Moreover, training must be ongoing, with opportunities for clinical supervision and informal consultation with colleagues as well as more formal in-service and continuing education.

Administrative policies within a service agency may support or interfere with the quality of clinical response afforded to infants and families. Is the practitioner's caseload a realistic size? Does the agency administration value outreach to difficult families? Are preventive efforts possible within the agency structure? Is time allowed for building a working alliance with a family and for long-term involvement with children and families?

The organization of services at the community level and beyond is also relevant to the clinical response. In some communities, health, education, and social services are organized in a way that makes it easy for practitioners to collaborate on behalf of a child and family. In other communities, even basic services do not exist or are not available for many families. Coping with the fragmentation of otherwise adequate services can sap the energies of parents and professionals alike. Coordinating services within the delivery system is a difficult and continuing task.

Policies of employers and governments are also part of the context in which clinical responses to babies and parents take place. Access to appropriate prenatal care, infant care leave, the provision of adequate income to families with young children, infant–toddler child care, housing policy, legislation concerning services for young children with disabilities, and allocation of health care resources are among the issues that define our society's current response to the needs of young children and families.

The detailed case reports in this volume allow the reader to see how elements of a clinical response interact. These reports tell us what manuals, protocols, guidelines, and even program evaluations and outcome measures cannot reveal: how one baby, one family, and one set of would-be helpers, with all their combined strengths, skills, resources, vulnerabilities, and histories, worked together for the healthy growth of the child. The contributors to this volume have recorded with care the language, behavior, emotional style, appearance, and other telling details about the infants and families with whom they have worked. They describe the opportunities and limits of their own work settings, their insights and perplexities as they make decisions, and their emotional responses as the work continues.

The three clusters of case reports in this volume may seem on the surface quite different from each other. The first cluster of reports concerns work with infants with disabilities and their families; the second cluster describes infants whose development is jeopardized by severe environmental stress. The behavioral problems of the infants described in the final cluster of three case reports may seem inconsequential in comparison. Yet in no case reported here would spontaneous resolution of the child's difficulties have been likely. Ignored or misunderstood, infants' and toddlers' "ordinary" sleep disturbances, fears of separation, and responses to marital conflict can jeopardize development and compromise seriously the nurturing relationship between children and parents.

A broad spectrum of child and family circumstances is presented in this volume in order to illustrate common themes as well as the range of clinical practice with infants, toddlers, and their families. The infants and toddlers described in these studies are all dealing with challenges common to the earliest years of life. The brief intervention that helps parents better understand their infant's experience and that frees them to find their own ways to support the child's development is an important, and effective, clinical response. Indeed, timely guidance and support may lessen the need for costly long-term interventions which must attempt to relieve major stress, repair damaged relationships, and provide intensive support to both child and family before development can move forward.

Each of the three clusters of case reports is introduced by material that emphasizes the elements of the clinical responses described in the reports: the conceptual framework, the unique needs of an individual child or family, the helping relationship, and the systems of care.

As readers of this book relate the rich particularities of each case report to the infants and families they themselves are working with or studying, they may also find it useful to keep in mind some overarching questions and themes.

1. What concern about the infant or toddler prompted the parent or parents to seek help, or motivated a professional to reach out to the family on behalf of the child?

2. Who decided that the development of the child was to some extent in jeopardy—that the child's situation or the relationship between parent and child was not likely to improve spontaneously?

3. What circumstances led each infant and family to the source of help described in the case report? What experiences had the family had with other professionals? (An interesting exercise is to imagine the family described in one case report appearing on the doorstep of an agency described in another report. How might the family have perceived and used services that were different from the ones they actually received? What issues might have received greater or lesser attention?)

4. What was the identified mission of the service program or setting described in each report? Were changes made in the agency's typical procedures to respond to the infant and family described?

5. How did the "facts of the case" emerge? To what extent did families and professionals reach a common understanding of the situation of infant and family?

6. What did parents, professionals, and involved others (referring sources, for example) expect to happen as a result of the clinical encounter? What sorts and degrees of positive change were seen as possible for child and/or family? How did people think change might be achieved?

7. What family members were available to be involved in an alliance on behalf of the young child's development? What was the actual role of extended family or of other potential informal sources of support?

8. What generic and discipline-specific skills did the primary intervenor bring to the work? What support was available from colleagues or supervisors within the agency?

8. To the extent that efforts from more than one professional or help from more than one agency was described, were these efforts coordinated or fragmented? What factors made a difference?

9. What was the time frame in which clinical work occurred? Were there particular circumstances that seemed either to speed up or delay prompt recognition of an infant's developmental problem? What factors seemed

to influence decisions about short- or long-term assessment and intervention?

Individually studied cases, carefully detailed and made available for scrutiny, form an important part of the knowledge base underlying all of the efforts of **ZERO TO THREE**/National Center for Clinical Infant Programs, sponsor of the *Clinical Infant Reports* series of which this volume is a part. We hope that they will be a useful resource for those who attempt to bring relief, offer comfort, and strengthen the adaptive capacities of infants, toddlers, and their families.

Part I:
Clinical Responses to Infants and Toddlers with Disabilities and Their Families

Sometimes conditions that lead to disabilities are recognized at birth. Sometimes concerns about an infant's health or development emerge over a period of months. A child may have a recognized "syndrome" or remain undiagnosed. However the disability of an infant or toddler becomes identified, parents, members of the extended family, health care providers, and other professionals are naturally concerned about the potential impact of the disability on the course of development.

The chapters by Fields, Blum, and Scharfman and by Blos and Davies remind us that appropriate clinical responses to young children with disabilities and their families must be complex responses. The presence of a defect or disability will undoubtedly affect the experience of the child and family; whether, or to what extent, a disability jeopardizes development is by no means certain. As the cases presented by these authors show us, hearing loss or neurological damage does not in itself predict the child's developmental course. Much more significant may be the support available to the infant to help him make the fullest possible use of his physical, cognitive, and emotional capacities.

Professionals who work with infants and toddlers with disabilities and their families are increasingly likely to acknowledge the central role of parents as the "constants" in their child's development; professional attention is increasingly likely, therefore, to focus on providing multifaceted support to the family rather than on simply "treatment" of an impairment or disability seen as residing within the child. The two chapters that follow suggest just how demanding a truly family-centered approach can be. They

3

also illustrate the far-reaching gains to be achieved by clinical responses that include the four elements described in the introduction to this volume.

A Conceptual Framework

Fields, Blum, and Scharfman and Blos and Davies describe therapeutic approaches to infants and families that are well grounded in psychodynamic and developmental conceptual frameworks. Blos and Davies, in fact, offer three distinct but complementary ways to understand the material they present—the psychodynamic, the behavioral, and the developmental. Both chapters illustrate the power that conceptual understanding gives to the worker as he or she chooses, and later evaluates, a therapeutic approach to the child and family.

Psychodynamic and developmental concepts help families, as well as professionals, to organize their experience. For example, if a parent can understand a young child's behavior as a communication, rather than as a manifestation of innate and immutable malevolence, the parent may be more likely to engage the child in dialogue, rather than simply to control behavior. If a parent can see a toddler's opposition to routines connected with hearing aids as a typical 2-year-old's response to threats to autonomy, the parent's experience of the child's behavior as "normal" may mitigate the burden of coping with difficult behavior.

Responsiveness to Individual Needs

The cases presented in these two chapters beautifully illustrate not only the uniqueness of each family likely to come to the attention of early intervention professionals but also the ways in which needs change, in intensity and in kind, over time. One issue of particular poignancy in work with infants, toddlers, and their families is that of balancing the needs of the family with those of the infant, at any given moment and over the course of the therapeutic relationship. Another challenge in this work, illustrated in both chapters, is the need to recognize and address the differences that may exist between the needs of the child and family as expressed by the parents and those needs as perceived by the worker. Both chapters describe the workers' conflicts and difficult choices, offering the reader valuable insights into the complexity of family-centered approaches. One also finds principles that can be used to guide individualized responses: for example, use the baby as the indicator of the care he is getting; speak or act so as to support, not undermine, the developing parent–child relationship.

Readers who are concerned about the provision of comprehensive services to infants and toddlers with disabilities and their families may find the discussion of mental health services in these two chapters particularly revealing. Blum, Fields, and Scharfman describe a service model specifically designed to address often unmet developmental needs of deaf infants and the emotional needs of their parents. Yet they recognize that parents bringing their infants for audiological diagnosis are seldom aware of the need for psychological intervention for themselves, their family, or their child. They suggest that a therapeutic approach that confirms and builds on parental strengths may not only be able to address emotional issues within the early intervention context but may also give parents a positive experience of mental health intervention on which to build in the future. In families such as the one described by Blos and Davies, the mental health needs of parents and children are often urgent, and offers of treatment not always accepted. Nevertheless, the worker's understanding of mental health issues allows him to remain aware of individual and family strengths despite the anxiety aroused by a mother's psychosis. He can be realistic about the limitations of the interventions acceptable to the family at a given time, and can also suggest what directions further work might take.

The Helping Relationship

The two chapters in this section illustrate the depth and complexity of the relationships that can develop between an infant–family professional and the members of a family with an infant with special needs. In the two service models presented, an infant–parent–worker triad forms the basis for a therapeutic alliance. Workers are also alert to the roles and needs of other family members, addressing these as appropriate.

Again, parent–professional relationship issues seem most vivid as workers define roles for themselves that will help to establish or nurture an alliance. Thus a therapist labors to communicate directly with a deaf mother, but refuses to accept the ultimately unhelpful role of therapist as surrogate caregiver for the infant. Another worker can be comfortable with a mother's introducing him as "the baby's therapist," different from a psychiatrist who might "dig into her mind and drive her crazy." He respects the mother's defensiveness and forms an alliance with her ability to transcend her own problems in order to care for her vulnerable infant.

The System of Care

Taken together, the two chapters in this section provide fascinating insights and raise provocative questions concerning the services available to infants and toddlers with special needs and their families. One wonders, first of all, how the lives of the parents described here might have been different had help been available early to address their own hearing loss or emotional problems, and to support their own parents. One also notes the difficulties, emotional and procedural, experienced by parents in securing financial assistance and access to specialized services. Will things be different as new legislation to expand and improve services to young children with disabilities is implemented?

A program's philosophy is reflected not only in intake procedures and treatment approaches but also in the use of staff, space, and materials, say Fields, Blum, and Scharfman. They offer a richly detailed model of how intervention within the context of a nursery setting works to address the developmental needs of deaf infants and the emotional needs of their parents. They also suggest that this model may be suitable for early preventive work with infants whose development may be in jeopardy for a variety of reasons. Ideally, a rich developmental nursery program would serve both children with disabilities and typically developing children, and offer support to their families as well.

Blos and Davies describe the many ironies and paradoxes involved in trying to provide comprehensive yet individualized care to infants and families within a complex medical setting. Staff of a neonatal intensive care unit, an infant psychiatry unit within a child psychiatry service, an emergency department, and an adult psychiatry clinic all see different aspects of the Emery family. Moreover, the Emerys perceive the various hospital services and personnel as very different entities, some helpful, some threatening. Not surprisingly, it is the strong personal relationship between one worker and the family that enables a substantial array of services to be provided in a reasonably coordinated manner. Comfortable, mutually respectful relationships among hospital staff in different departments and between hospital and community-based practitioners also work to the benefit of children and family.

1

Mental Health Intervention with Very Young Children and Their Parents: A Model Based on the Infant Deaf

Barbara Fields, M.A., M.S.W., Elsa J. Blum, Ph.D., Helen Scharfman, M.S.W.

Introduction

Recent research has addressed the importance of early childhood development for later functioning and findings have suggested the need for early intervention for infants at risk. The handicap of severe to profound deafness can be viewed as placing the deaf infant at risk for less than optimal development (Rothstein, 1975), but does not inevitably result in as poor an outcome as the literature on the status of the deaf adult might indicate. In fact, variability of achievement levels and social adjustment within the deaf population suggests that the handicap of

Acknowledgments. The authors wish to acknowledge the important contributions of Dr. Eleanor Galenson who was initially director of the Infant/Parent Nursery at the Lexington Center for Mental Health Services, and who supervised the cases described. Staff members and volunteers who have worked with the authors in this nursery over the years also contributed considerably to the development of the ideas presented in this paper. In particular, we would like to acknowledge the work of Diana Silber, M.S.W.

9

deafness per se is not solely responsible for the limitations so often attributed to deaf children and adults. Our own observations support the idea that other factors besides the auditory deficit significantly influence the course of development and later functioning in deaf children, and we propose that some of these factors are potentially malleable and accessible to early intervention.

The Impact of Deafness on the Developmental Process

Deaf infants are, of course, vulnerable due to direct consequences of the auditory deficit, most notably in relation to communication and the effects of delayed language on other aspects of the developmental process. The impact of congenital deafness on social and emotional development is less obvious but most likely affects these processes at their earliest levels. Precursors of what will later become linguistic conversation emerge within the context of developing object relations, and distortions in one sphere significantly affect the other. For example, modifications in the deaf infant's response may intrude upon the rhythm and tempo of the prelinguistic dialogue described by Stern (1974a), adversely affecting important aspects of early reciprocity. Weil (1978) notes the mother's critical role as facilitator of preverbal forms of communication. Her description of the mother as both stimulating and being stimulated by the child's vocalization raises the question of how early mother–child interactions are altered when the deaf infant is unable to be aurally stimulated, then, some months later, ceases babbling. Because the usual maternal response is not elicited, nor the normal maternal overture responded to, the parent–child relationship is modified in subtle but meaningful ways. Additionally, the mother's voice cannot act as an organizer to bring the infant to a state of quiet alertness, to focus the baby's attention, or to draw it back when it strays from the interaction occurring between them. The absence of a primary distance perceptor, an insurmountable obstacle to the deaf child's ability to maintain contact when the parent is not visible, along with the lack of auditory memory traces in the establishment of self and object representations, undoubtedly influence the separation–individuation process in ways that are not yet altogether clear. The course and quality of self–object differentiation, evolving symbolic capacities (Drucker, 1979), and integrative functions (Fields, 1979), are affected as well.

Of equal significance is the alteration of the parent–child relationship due to the parents' affective response to the child's deficit. Naturally, parental responses differ, but among the most common are feelings of guilt, depression, anger, often disguised, and a sense of injury and loss surrounding the realization that the child is not intact (Solnit and Stark, 1961; Rothstein, 1975). Marital stress, family disruption, and withdrawal from the child frequently result as each parent tries to cope with his or her grief. Such parental responses further exacerbate the child's handicap by limiting activation and enrichment of nonauditory, as well as auditory modalities, and by communication of depressed and/or angry affect. Since this often occurs during the period when developmental processes are particularly sensitive to maternal distress, the especially attuned parenting required for optimal development in these children may not be available. Thus, the deaf infant, who needs more than the usual degree of maternal involvement to facilitate both affective and cognitive functions, may actually receive less. Other authors (Freedman, Cannady, and Robinson, 1971; Rainer, 1976; Rothstein, 1979) have suggested that determinants of characteristics usually attributed to the adult deaf population may be found in early mother–child relationships. While we agree that maternal reactions to the impairment play a large role in the formation of the deaf child's later personality and functioning, the influence of the deficit itself cannot be minimized.

Deaf parents' reactions to their child's deficit may be somewhat different, more ambivalent and less intense than those of hearing parents. For deaf parents, the birth of a hearing impaired child is neither a complete surprise nor totally undesired. While for numerous reasons these parents may hope for an intact child, many also express a wish for a child like themselves with whom they can share a close affective and communicative relationship. The fear of rejection by a hearing child is also an issue for some deaf parents. Despite these differences, many of the responses described above are common to both deaf and hearing parents whose child is found to be deaf.

Because educational institutions for the deaf are primarily concerned with the educational and audiological implications of deafness, parents tend to view their child's deficit within this framework rather than from a more comprehensive developmental perspective. This problem is compounded by differing educational approaches to congenital deafness that parents encounter, which contribute to their general sense of helpless confusion about what is available and optimal for their child. Under these typical circumstances, the special developmental needs of deaf infants and the emotional needs of their parents are generally unmet.

A Parent–Infant Intervention Program

In an attempt to address those issues, the therapeutic nursery at the Lexington School for the Deaf, New York City, was established in 1974 as an early intervention and research setting for deaf infants below the age of 3 (with no other handicapping conditions), and their parents. As such, it augmented existing audiological and educational programs for this population and became the mental health component of infant services at Lexington.

Nursery goals encompass what we view as critical and highly interrelated aspects of affective and cognitive development. These aspects are: a deeper understanding of a developmental process impinged upon by severe to profound deafness; and the facilitation of a more salutary unfolding of cognitive, communicative, and interpersonal capacities in deaf infants. The reciprocal nature of the mother–child relationship forms the basis of our theoretical and clinical perspective and our utilization of the tripartite model of intervention based on Mahler's (1968, 1979) work with psychotic children. In Mahler's design, the therapist worked together with mother and child (hence the term *tripartite*), with the goal of enabling a corrective symbiotic experience from which separation-individuation could then proceed. Although the deaf infants attending the Lexington nursery are not psychotic, Mahler's model was readily adapted to our purpose. As in the Mahler design, mother and child are seen together in treatment, the therapist becoming a bridge between them. In our case, however, the aim is to generally enrich a parent–child relationship jeopardized by the circular impact of congenital deafness and parental response to the handicapped child. Mahler's model was initially adapted to a nursery setting by Galenson (1984) at the Albert Einstein College of Medicine and later modified by her for the Lexington nursery (Galenson, Miller, Kaplan, and Rothstein, 1979; Galenson, Kaplan, Miller, and Rothstein, 1979). In the application of this model we have attempted to integrate our expanding knowledge of difficulties common to most deaf infants and their parents with a clinical understanding of the individual parent's and child's needs and capacities.

Intake

The therapeutic process begins with the first family contact, usually around the time of the initial diagnosis of deafness at the Lexington Hearing and Speech Center where the child's hearing is carefully assessed and closely followed.[1] This is a critical period for families. Many months of anxious concern usually precede the diagnosis; marital distress along with parental withdrawal from each other and from the impaired child frequently begins with the earliest suspicions of deafness. Siblings of the deaf infant are also jeopardized by parental reactions to the prolonged crisis.

Intake interviews are carried out by a nursery therapist, if possible by the therapist who will work with the parents and child, and involve all significant family members, sometimes including extended family. Assessment includes information gathering about parental histories, the marriage, and the family unit. Each parent's relationship to his or her deaf child as well as to other children in the family is explored. Psychological strengths and areas of conflict are assessed and beginning dynamic understanding is formulated. The child's developmental status is evaluated by history and observation with emphasis on the unfolding development of the drives, ego, and object relatedness. When indicated, the therapist begins to explore with the parent the possibility of financial aid from federal and state governments. Along with assessment, this initial phase of treatment has the aim of acquainting families with our service and helping them become aware of their need for intervention by beginning to explore the impact of the child's deafness on his or her development, on themselves, and on their family.

The tendency of many parents to deny both the extent of their reactions and the need for mental health services is a core issue of this early treatment phase. In contrast to

---

[1]Careful and ongoing evaluation of hearing loss and decisions about the effectiveness of various hearing aids are crucial to the treatment of hearing impairments.

most patients who, however resistant, actively seek psycho-therapeutic help, parents of deaf infants bringing their child for audiological diagnosis are usually unaware of the need for psychological intervention for themselves, their family, or their child. Parents require sensitive assistance in viewing intervention in a positive light. They need particularly to experience therapeutic intervention as addressed to adaptive parental attributes, as well as to those aspects of personality which might adversely affect their child's potential. Earliest therapeutic efforts thus support the parents' ability to work through an extraordinary and critical life event, rather than emphasizing existing or incipient pathology.

Treatment

Parents and children attend two, one-and-a-half-hour nursery sessions each week, each pair with its own therapist. At any one session, there are usually two to four infant–parent dyads in the nursery. The room is large and airy, furnished with a variety of age-appropriate toys and play equipment, and a comfortable sitting area. We are fortunate in having an L-shaped room that affords more chance for seclusion than is ordinarily available in a nursery setting, offering areas where parent, child, and therapist can work relatively undisturbed. Nursery therapists are aware of each other's clinical needs and often arrange before a nursery session to assure the privacy of a particular therapist and dyad. Since the demands of an infant or toddler often limit opportunities for individual work with parents, when indicated, another nursery therapist can include the child with her own dyad. An adjoining office is also used at times when more privacy is needed. The advantages and disadvantages of treatment within a nursery setting will be explored in the conclusion of this paper as one of the issues arising from the kind of intervention we describe.

Treatment takes place on a variety of levels addressing both the immediate needs of the family in crisis and the longer range developmental and therapeutic goals previously described. Since the emphasis of treatment depends in each case on the unique needs and capacities of the specific dyad, different but generally interrelated clinical modes are utilized. Where parents can be engaged in the exploration of their less conscious thoughts and feelings and motivations for behavior, intervention addresses these issues, especially as they impinge upon their child's development. When parents do not seem capable of engaging in this kind of self-examination, a counseling approach, providing a supportive climate for the expression of feelings, and developmental guidance, including the clarification of issues related to deafness, has been a more central feature of treatment. Generally, our work encompasses a range of interventions within each case, but usually one mode predominates as the case material presented later in the paper will illustrate.

The therapist–parent relationship is perhaps the major element in tripartite work. The parent's growing attachment to the therapist and the alliance that develops between them, paves the way for the long-term, continued exploration, expression, and interpretation of parental feelings and ideas. Some of the deaf mothers were daughters of deaf parents, but many had hearing parents. In the case of deaf mothers with hearing parents, the women may have to some extent been deprived of positive and stable relationships with their own parents. In such cases, the formation of a strong, therapeutic bond becomes a particularly critical treatment issue. The empathic milieu created by the therapist also provides an often much needed maternal kind of nurturing, which, because of deficits in their early experience, seems especially significant for deaf mothers. Hearing mothers as well may initially require a nurturing relationship, when the extended family, frequently in a state of turmoil following the diagnosis of deafness, is unable to offer the family meaningful support. Even when the family situation is more positive following diagnosis, parental feelings of shame and narcissistic injury, both before and after diagnosis, tend to interfere with relationships within the extended family; both affective and realistic burdens may be overwhelming. While dependent needs are often gratified, however, especially in the earlier phase of treatment, the ultimate therapeutic goal is to help parents achieve an understanding about themselves that leads to more independent functioning.

The presence of child and parent together in treatment offers the opportunity for parental identification with the therapist's positive regard for the child; the parent may come to believe on an emotional level, as well as intellectually, that the defective child is indeed lovable and worthy of attention and acceptance by others. By observing the therapist and interacting with her, the parent begins to internalize both the therapist's modes of relating to the child and her ideas and attitudes about development. Through modeling and counseling, and less consciously, through identification with the therapist, the parent can become more appropriately and consistently responsive to his or her deaf child.

A number of aspects of tripartite intervention can be illustrated by the description of our approach to two typically encountered issues. The first concerns the application of hearing aids, which, of course, is specific to deaf infants and their parents. The second concerns separation anxiety, which is an issue for all young children but appears to be heightened in deaf infants.

The process of being fitted for and becoming acclimatized to hearing aids usually progresses in tandem with intake and beginning nursery participation and involves a number of procedures. First, plastic impressions of the child's internal ear structure are used to make ear molds which are connected to one of two types of hearing aids. Without exception, the children at the Lexington nursery wear ear-level aids.[2] These are the commonly observed skin-tinted hearing aids worn behind the ear. Whichever type of hearing aid is utilized, the child needs to become accustomed to the insertion of the ear mold, in the beginning often many times daily. As might be imagined, this insertion frequently elicits varying degrees of oppositional response on the part of the child, causing further strain in the parent–child relationship. The child also must become acclimated to increasing amounts of aural stimulation. In this regard, it is important to mention that hearing aids approximate but are not equivalent to normal hearing, nor do aids bestow hearing adequate enough for the normal acquisition of language.

The process of being fitted for and becoming acclimatized to hearing aids, referred to in the literature and in this paper as "aiding" or "the aiding process," seems to be viewed by most parents, consciously and unconsciously, as both a cure for the impairment and a clear public symbol of the defect. Fantasies about the redemptive and restorative powers of the hearing aids abound and often serve resistance to addressing developmental issues and parental reactions. Thus, issues around aiding bring into sharp focus parental feelings about the deficit itself. For deaf parents, their own early feelings about the use of hearing aids, often stemming from unpleasant experiences associated with their first school years and separation from their mothers, are reawakened. Part of the work in this area

---

[2]The other type of aid is known as a body aid, and amplification is enclosed in a box worn on the chest. While body aids are considered by many to be old fashioned and cumbersome, some audiologists believe they provide a greater amount of amplification for children with certain types of hearing loss than is possible with ear-level aids.

consists of educating parents about the use of hearing aids. A primary aim, however, is to help parents distinguish between appropriate responses to the reality of the aiding process and those responses that are determined by less conscious thoughts and feelings. For example, a parent who consciously wants his or her child to be aided may handle the process ambivalently because aiding precludes denying the infant's deafness. In the same way, throughout the course of treatment, parents are helped to explore the interweaving of reality based issues with deeper, more conflicted responses. Where parental limitations make this kind of exploration impossible, support for parents and therapeutic work with the child nonetheless proceed during the aiding process.

Although some aspects of parental responses to situations like the aiding process can, and perhaps should, be worked through individually with the parent, tripartite treatment plays an important role in its focus on the interchanges occurring between parent and child. For example, parents who are ambivalent or fearful about the application of hearing aids, or who find themselves in a distressing struggle with their child, are helped by therapeutic intervention aimed at supporting both members of the dyad during aiding. Play with the child around the aiding process also helps parents understand issues which their child is attempting to master. Such play may be especially important for deaf parents who are helped to rework issues related to their own early aiding through observing or becoming actively engaged in their child's activities. The child's activity also can become a catalyst for parental expression of feelings surrounding their child's handicap, and in the case of deaf parents, their own deficit as it affects ideas about themselves and their child.

While separation–individuation (Mahler, 1974; Mahler, Pine, and Bergman, 1975) is a universal process, for many reasons, the deaf infant's response to separation is

heightened and prolonged. Parental reactions to this vulnerability may range from denial that the child is anxious
to an inability to allow age-appropriate distancing. We
have found that most, if not all, parents need guidance in
understanding their child's reaction to separation and
fears of object loss, as well as specific issues related to deafness that may intensify such concerns. In a tripartite setting, aspects of the child's and parent's response to separation are repeatedly brought to parental attention in
relation to the child's nursery activity. For instance, parents of a deaf child who often left him with unfamiliar
people and who had many transient visitors from the country where they were born, were helped to understand the
meaning of these experiences for the child by the therapist's observations of his behavior, play, and mood in their
association with developmental issues and real events in
family life. Through these observations, built up gradually
over the course of treatment, the parents began to understand their child's response to separation related themes,
as well as their ambivalent reactions which affected not
only their child's development but their own struggle for
independence from their respective families. Thus, when
parent and child are both present in treatment, frequently,
the child's behaviors and reactions can be used as illustrative data to link developmental issues, family practices,
events in current home life, and parental history, high-
lighting for the parent the interplay of forces which shape
their child's development. Over a period of time, a way of
thinking about development is established which can be
integrated by the parents and employed in understanding
and addressing future developmental events. Often elements of parental reaction to issues like separation must
be explored in relation to their own history, family, and
cultural values, and as responses to their deaf child. In
addition, young deaf children need ample opportunity to

play out a range of separation-related themes, for example, in relation to fear of loss of a body part and product as well as loss of mother. We often suggest concrete, practical ways for parents to help their deaf toddlers anticipate and master actual and psychological separation, and communicate about past and future events; for example, a book of photographs depicting such things as parental activities away from home, relatives, family outings, nursery peers, and therapists. All these approaches are employed within a given nursery session and over the course of treatment. Similarly, emphasis shifts periodically between parent and child, according to emerging needs of both, and as conflicts arise or achieve a degree of resolution.

Naturally, in our work with children play is a major therapeutic mode. Besides encouraging the unfolding of manipulative, perceptual, communicative, and social skills, play is employed as a means of mastering conflict, typical developmental strains, and problems specific to or exacerbated by deafness. Since both sensorimotor and semisymbolic play of deaf infants and toddlers often appears meager or limited, much of our own work involves offering the children opportunities for sustained explorative and imaginative play, and following their lead, helping them to extend play ideas. Because it is so difficult to sustain and/or elaborate the young deaf child's play through language, a great deal of ingenuity is required on the therapist's part to help the child maintain interest and focus. The development of reciprocity in play and the understanding that the child's activity conveys meaning to others is especially significant for these children. Close attention to the child's postural, gestural, and affective cues aids the therapist in these tasks and in guiding and elaborating play ideas in concordance with developmental needs and interests.

Particular sensitivity is required with children whose play may be inhibited due to conflict. The following illustration provides an example of how the therapist was able to extend the play of such a child making it available as a therapeutic modality.

> Nicky, a 22-month-old toddler, was having many battles for control with his mother, along with sleep and separation difficulties, and seemed hampered in his ability to use play for mastery or in the service of ameliorating developmental stress. One day, when Nicky began switching a light on and off, the therapist suggested that she and Nicky's mother pretend to sleep when Nicky turned the lights off and wake up when he turned them on. With delighted smiles, Nicky stayed at his game, returning to it for some part of each nursery session for many weeks, permitting the therapist to verbally link his activity with issues related to autonomy and separation, which she and Nicky's mother had been discussing.

This brief vignette highlights a number of salient features of our work. First, an understanding of developmental processes in conjunction with psychoanalytic principles, allows the therapist to utilize and translate symbolically expressed concerns into active, reciprocal play around conflicted issues. Of particular importance in tripartite treatment, developmental issues not only need to be appreciated by the therapist, but conveyed to the parent in ways that on some level clarify the nature of the conflict and the interventions employed. By these means, the child's behavioral expressions of conflict, and the largely inchoate ideas and feelings generated by internal stress and strivings can be organized in ways that make at least some of their content both understandable to the parent and available to the child for mastery. Additionally, the therapist must be attuned enough to the child to help him or her transform an essentially egocentric activity into one with shared communicative value. Since preverbal forms of communication, as well as language per se, may be compromised by congenital deafness, play is a particularly important vehicle for shared communication with significant others. The therapist's or parent's contingent and invested response to the child's activity and indication of intentionality can lend real meaning to the interactions occurring around and within play, and promote in the deaf child feelings of efficacy necessary for ego and cognitive growth.

With deaf children the facilitation of reciprocity in play is often burdened by didactic concerns on the part of the parents. Both hearing and deaf parents tend to feel that if their deaf child is "playing" he or she is not "learning," and frequently view play as wasting precious time that could be used in teaching language to their child. Paradoxically, the parents' anxious and often intrusive demands for speech or sign language not only create tension between parent and child, but also effectively end a play episode, adversely affecting the construction of symbols by pulling the child away from activity which builds meaning. We feel our task here is to help parents find a balance between the expression of their quite natural anxieties about signed and/or spoken word production, and allowing these concerns to become an overriding issue interfering with true communication and play. Parents also need help in understanding the relationship of word production to broader aspects of language development, and in recognizing play as an essential ingredient of the meaning making process underlying developing symbolic functions. Because didactic concerns usually take precedence over a more playful kind of exchange between parent and child, reciprocal play is also encouraged with the intent that some of the sheer pleasure and fun inherent in playing with one's child will promote the sense of mutual delight, good will, and intimacy that shared, playful activity imparts.

Case Illustrations

The case discussions that follow illustrate some of the therapeutic possibilities within the tripartite structure of the nursery. The emphasis in each case is different; the clinical work is molded by the specific needs and capacities of each parent and child. The first case will describe our work with Jeff and his hearing mother and will highlight the integration of psychodynamically oriented therapy and developmental guidance that became the predominant treatment mode. The case of Tommy and his mother, who is profoundly deaf, necessitated a somewhat different approach in which supportive, reparative measures with both members of the dyad predominated. In both cases, work with the children played a major therapeutic role.

JEFF

Jeff entered the nursery at 18 months of age. He is the first-born child of Mr. and Mrs. J, both of whom are hearing, as are all the other members of their immediate families. When Jeff was 4 to 6 months of age, his parents began to suspect that something might be wrong with their child. Over the next few months, they contacted two pediatricians but, as often happens, both helped to reinforce the J's' denial by reassuring them that children do not always respond to all sounds. When Jeff was 1½ years old and still not responding to his name, the J's finally brought him to Lexington where he was found to have a profound bilateral sensory neural hearing loss. This elapsed time between the parents' first suspicion and the certainty of the final diagnosis delayed the beginning of aiding, auditory training, and entry into the nursery.

Mr. and Mrs. J were high-school sweethearts from working-class backgrounds who married after graduation and soon had Jeff. During our initial evaluation period we found them to be empathic, caring, and responsive parents. They enjoyed playing with Jeff and provided him with varied and rich verbal, kinesthetic, and emotional experiences. Even profoundly deaf children can derive meaning from lip movements, facial expressions, gesture, and, once hearing aids are being used, from auditory input as well. Jeff's parents intuitively seemed to understand the importance of establishing both a nonverbal and verbal dialogue with their son.

Mrs. J, a warm sweet young woman, generally seemed to know instinctively what was right for her child. As a youngster she had enjoyed playing with dolls and now seemed to fully enjoy this real live doll. She was, however, when we met, a very dependent young woman, lacking in self-confidence, who found it difficult to separate from her own mother or to do anything on her own away from home. Little was known about her father who had died when she was about 4 years old. Mr. J, also warm and caring despite a "macho" manner, evidenced little ambition to further his education or to leave his lower-level, blue-collar job.

The J's lived in a small apartment in Mrs. J's mother's home, the same house where Mrs. J had lived all her life, within walking distance of Mr. J's family as well. The J's felt that they were treated like children by their respective families, since Mr. J's family controlled their bankbooks, and both families were constantly interfering in their private affairs. They were also often unhappy recipients of well-meaning family advice about raising Jeff. This was especially traumatic for them during the diagnosis and evaluation of his deafness. Some family members suggested shopping around for many more diagnoses; still others suggested possible operations, while others assured the parents that Jeff would probably outgrow the handicap by the time he was 5. The J's, overwhelmed by self-doubt and guilt, were constantly wondering whether they were doing what was best for their child.

Jeff was a bright, cheerful, friendly, and energetic toddler when he came to the nursery. His parents rarely had any difficulty understanding him for he used many gestures and a large variety of facial expressions. When we met Jeff he also had an expressive oral vocabulary of four words, *Mamy, Dada, up,* and *hot.* He was still on the bottle and toilet training had not yet begun. In the nursery Jeff mirrored his parents' responsiveness by displaying an unusual degree of empathy toward his nursery peers. He was especially gentle and solicitous of younger children, and though he was not old enough to take part in any kind of reciprocal play, Jeff watched his peers closely, often imitated them, and appeared to enjoy their presence.

While separation is a particularly salient issue for many 18-month-old toddlers, for Jeff the problem was exacerbated by his deafness. Although he was comfortable with both children and adults, his mother was obviously a special person whom he kept well within reach and sight. He found it difficult to tolerate even the momentary separation imposed by closing his eyes, and became easily upset if a T-shirt or sweater were not pulled over his head with great haste. He did not yet have hearing aids, and although he was in tactile contact with his mother, this was not enough to alleviate his anxiety. Mrs. J encouraged Jeff's close attachment; he was never left with a baby-sitter, was included in all of the J's' activities, and slept in their bedroom. In the nursery, Mrs. J was usually close to Jeff and actively participated in all his activities, but in her eagerness to help, she often prevented Jeff from solving tasks on his own.

One of the therapist's initial functions within the tripartite nursery setting was to develop a supportive relationship with Mrs. J, enabling her to differentiate her own thoughts and feelings from the sometimes irrational, intrusive attitudes of the extended families. She began to trust her own judgment and gradually gained some assurance of her own competence as a parent upon whom special demands would be made. She was given the therapist's home telephone number, and, although she never used it, seemed reassured by the therapist's availability. In response to her myriad questions, factual information about deafness was offered to help Mrs. J understand the reality of Jeff's condition and prognosis. During those first few months, the therapist accompanied Mrs. J in her quest for state aid,[3] often a humiliating and debilitating experience. The therapist was also present during two other traumatic events, when the initial ear mold impressions were made and when hearing aids were given to Jeff. The latter was a profound emotional experience for Mrs. J, for it not only reinforced, on a concrete level, the diagnosis of deafness, but poignantly symbolized the reality of the deficit. At the same time, the hearing aids offered the hope of magical restitution and when Jeff turned toward a sound for the first time after the audiologist fitted the aids and clapped her hands, Mrs. J burst into uncontrollable sobs.

During the next months as a positive therapeutic alliance developed, treatment was gradually directed toward Mrs. J's difficulty in separating from Jeff. While multidetermined and in some respects similar to other parents' perceptions of their handicapped children as particularly dependent and vulnerable, Mrs. J's tendency to infantilize Jeff stemmed to a great extent from her own particular dynamics and conflicts. Gradually it became clear that her relationship with Jeff replicated many aspects of her relationship with her own mother. She became aware that her mother's need to keep her closely tied and dependent was reciprocally related to her own dependency and self-doubt. While angry at being infantilized, at the same time she had more than ordinary difficulty in becoming an independent young adult. As Mrs. J began to separate from her mother and to function more autonomously in her

---

[3]If income requirements are met, New York State reimburses some of the costs incurred due to a handicapping condition.

own life, she was able to allow Jeff to function more independently also. She no longer turned to her mother or in-
laws for support or advice, and began to rely on her own
judgment. Previously afraid, she now began to drive a car,
and toward the end of the first treatment year she was able
to move to a new apartment far from the extended family.
These changes reflected the insights gained from the exploration of dynamic issues and the positive transference
to the therapist who was viewed as both supportive and as
promoting more autonomous functioning. Jeff, in turn,
became able to tolerate increasing periods of time out of
visual contact with his mother. He used her less as a facilitator and seemed secure in the knowledge that she was
available if needed. At home Jeff was given his own bedroom and weaning was achieved. The latter had been discussed for many months, but it was only after the attendant
work on separation that it was quickly accomplished.

At about 25 months Jeff was easily toilet trained with
little pressure and apparently eager compliance. About
one month after toilet training was well on its way, Jeff
began to resist having his ear molds inserted. He verbal-
ized that they hurt and struggled whenever his mother
attempted to aid him. Increasingly upset, Mrs. J forced
Jeff to lie immobile while she inserted the molds and
placed the aids behind his ears, which seemed to intensify
his resistance. Considering this from a developmental
viewpoint, we realized that therapeutic efforts directed toward promoting autonomy had indeed succeeded, so
much so that Jeff was now engaged in a struggle with his
parents. Perhaps experiencing aiding as an intrusion, and
particularly resenting being placed in a submissive supine
position while the ear molds were inserted, he was rebel-
ling, proclaiming his separateness and individuality in typical 2-year-old fashion. After weighing the consequences of
a temporary loss of acoustical input, we counseled Jeff's
parents against the use of hearing aids for a few days in

order to allow the struggle to abate. Because the struggle for autonomy was coincident with toilet training, we also suggested that all toileting efforts be put aside unless explicitly initiated by Jeff. Finally, because Mr. J was not involved in this conflict and because Jeff was beginning to identify with him, we encouraged Mr. J to take part in the aiding process. We advised against placing Jeff in a supine position while aiding him since he seemed to equate this position with submission and loss of autonomy. We also suggested aiding Jeff in front of a mirror, a three-way one if possible, so that he could see his ears and observe the process.

For the first few days that Jeff was without hearing aids he seemed happy and relieved. He ran around pretending to hear sounds, however, suggesting he missed the input. For example, he would point to the fire alarm bell/light in the classroom which was silent, point to his ear and shake his head as if to tell us he heard it. During those days and for some weeks afterward, Jeff showed a great interest in other children's hearing aids and watched closely when they were aided. He also frequently initiated play with our play molds and aids, aiding dolls, his mother, and the therapist, just as he had during the initial aiding process many months before. Finally, by repeating the aiding process many times over as the active, rather than the passive participant, and by discharging through play some of the anger apparently aroused by the event, Jeff was able once again to accept his hearing aids. He continued to assert his autonomy by controlling the time and place of aiding, which his parents sensitively allowed.

As the struggle for autonomy seemed to abate, Jeff's anger diminished. This partial resolution of the ambivalence inherent in the struggle for autonomy permitted better consolidation of object constancy (Mahler et al., 1975). This, in turn, made brief separations from his mother more tolerable, although regressions in his level of play and capacity for focused attention still often occurred in her absence. While Jeff had manifested social interest in his peers at a young age, it was only when he began to distance himself from his mother that he actively sought them out in play. Jeff also now showed a change in his relationship to the therapist, relating to her as a special person. He looked for her when coming to the nursery, tried to say her name, and wanted to share his activities with her as well as with his mother. Jeff's behavior suggested that one manifestation of a child's burgeoning psychological separation from his mother may be a newly acquired availability for other relationships.

Within a few months Jeff began to display a new level of symbolic capacity. His play took on an entirely new character, incorporating sequential pretend play for the first time. He began to accept the reading of picture books, an activity previously avoided. He also used puzzles, learned colors, categorized shapes, and started to count. Language development markedly improved, with Jeff progressing from one-word communications to four- and five-word sentences. At age 3 Jeff made an adequate transition to the Lexington preschool, gradually tolerating separation from his mother and maintaining the developmental gains he had made in the nursery.

Once Jeff had left the infant nursery Mrs. J began to meet weekly with the therapist on an individual basis. She continued to show overall improvement in functioning and in understanding the relationship of her past history to current life events and was able to deal with her mother's death in an appropriate manner, without undue regression. She moved toward the resolution of some of the painful conflicts related to her child's deafness including residual feelings of guilt and narcissistic injury. While these reactions emerged quite early in treatment they proved to encompass complex and multidetermined issues which required working through over a long period of time. The early tripartite nursery treatment appeared to have achieved its immediate goal of preventing serious developmental distortion and served as a preliminary to individual treatment, the need for which might otherwise not have been recognized.

TOMMY

The second case to be discussed, that of Tommy, reflects some similarities and differences in our treatment approach. We began work with Tommy, the only child of first-generation deaf parents, when he was 10 months old. Because of the genetic history of deafness, Tommy was examined at a university hospital at 3½ months. He was assessed as hearing impaired but the degree of deafness was not ascertained. Six months later, Tommy was brought to Lexington where unaided tests revealed a bilateral, moderate to severe sensory neural impairment.

Despite this relatively moderate loss, at 10 months Tommy seemed like a child with a more severe deficit. He rarely vocalized, showed little interest in sounds, and made minimal use of his residual hearing. Oral language was provided by hearing members of the large, extended, maternal and paternal families, none of whom signed. Tommy's parents were not skilled orally and communicated primarily through American Sign Language (ASL). Yet, their use of signing rarely included Tommy. Thus, the lack of signed communication with their son perhaps reflected early prohibitions and ensuing conflicts around the use of sign language in their own lives, as well as the depression that seemed to accompany the diagnosis of Tommy's deafness.

Beyond this, Mrs. T was unable to provide a consistently nurturing environment for her son, a limitation that seemed closely linked to events in her own early life. These included a history of early deprivation due to maternal depression as well as a later, prolonged separation from her mother at 4 years of age. The dual and interrelated factors of maternal depression and her own profound hearing loss no doubt had serious implications for Mrs. T's early development. As an adult, Mrs. T was an attractive young woman who, over the course of treatment, became increasingly related, competent, and forthright. When we first met, however, she tended to be infantilized by her family, who expected very little of their only daughter and acted as her interpreters to the hearing world. Mrs. T also manifested a limited capacity for empathy and self-reflection, and tended to deal with ideas and events concretely. Tommy's father, a gentle young man, was an active participant in his son's development and daily care. His relationship with Tommy was loving and involved, although marred by a teasing quality that also suffused Mrs. T's relationship with their son.

Like many 10-month-old infants, Tommy came to us very tied to bottle and pacifier. Although barely crawling, this seemed largely a matter of performance rather than competence since his general development was within normal limits. His emotional responses ranged from occasional playful engagement to a more frequent solemnity that over the course of the first few months became his predominant mood. Tommy's level of motor activity, his initiative, and general interest in exploration, were subject to the same variations.

While quite familiar with many members of his close-knit, extended family, Tommy clearly preferred his mother. His increasingly anxious attempts, however, to be close to her and keep her in sight were met by a marked lack of empathy and denial of Tommy's response to separation. On a more profound level such responses reflected the basic lack of mutuality and reciprocity that seemed to pervade the relationship between Tommy and his mother. Mrs. T rarely responded to Tommy's clearly expressed needs and cues. When Tommy put his head in his mother's lap, her arms remained passively at her sides. She was rigid in her prohibitions of oral and other age-appropriate explorations, both of Tommy's own body and the outside world. Early reciprocal games involving tactile and kinesthetic experience were few and presaged Mrs. T's later reluctance to participate in more advanced play activities. In addition, both Tommy and his mother seemed passive in seeking out experience. If a ball rolled under a couch and Tommy wanted it (indicated by leaning forward, looking at the ball and his mother), Mrs. T did not respond. Tommy's reaction mirrored his mother's. He sat inert until the object was retrieved by someone else.

The family's treatment proceeded along three major lines: the development of the therapeutic bond with Mrs. T, treatment directed toward the dyad, and interventions with Tommy that did not require Mrs. T's direct participation. These interventions were, of course, fluid and interrelated, reflecting the special needs of the mother–child pair and our increasing understanding of the dynamics of their relationship.

As the therapist initially knew no sign language and Mrs. T used little oral language, the most crucial issue in building a therapeutic relationship was the lack of a shared communicative mode. It is difficult to convey the sense of limited relatedness that pervaded beginning attempts to communicate with Mrs. T. Although the therapist tried never to pretend to understand when she did not, Mrs. T clearly did just that, even though in time she made heroic efforts to reach her therapist and to understand her communications. Additionally, as the child of a hearing mother, Mrs. T had virtually no mother tongue to share with either the therapist or her son. A mutual language was sorely needed to link Mrs. T's linguistic experience to that of her therapist and child, with all the affective resonance such a connection implies. While it immediately became clear that a shared communicative mode was essential to treatment, the therapist's persistence in communicating without the aid of a family or outside interpreter, even prior to her learning sign language, paved the way for the formation of a therapeutic bond. During the course of treatment a shared language was built up through gestures and pantomime, interspersed with simple, concrete oral phrases. American Sign Language and elements of Signed English were added as the therapist learned these languages, both to establish as wide a range of communication as possible, and because the endorsement of sign served as a core of acceptance and approval. To some extent, Mrs. T also became better able to express herself orally.

But the gap to be bridged involved more than communication, for in our work with Mrs. T we noted a striking polarity. On the one hand there was a core of deprivation related to the precarious nature of her early life as the deaf child of a depressed, withdrawn mother, and on the other, ongoing infantilization as an adult. The auditory deficit and dysfunctional development patterns combined to impede both Mrs. T's own development and undermine maternal capacities, with negative effects for Tommy's development as well. Our understanding of these issues naturally influenced our therapeutic approach, and interventions aimed at Mrs. T were generally directed toward unresolved developmental issues, most specifically addressing the dual tasks of enriching aspects of object relations and reinforcing the more autonomous features of personality.

Our first task with Mrs. T centered around facilitating a shift from her nearly total dependence on her family to increasing reliance on the nursery and therapist. The issue of extended family participation, like many other interventions, was not explicitly addressed. For example, the therapist never urged Mrs. T to come alone, and for a period of time at least one family member always joined her. Over the first few months of treatment, however, the family was gradually but purposely assigned a background role, and after about three-and-a-half months Mrs. T first drove to the nursery herself, with Tommy. We do not know if this decision to come alone was self-initiated or proposed by family members. It is possible that because of the relationship established during intake and the earliest phase of treatment, the family felt more secure and through overt and/or covert messages facilitated Mrs. T's more independent functioning.

Concomitant with the partial shift away from her family, Mrs. T turned to the therapist with the expectation that the latter would assume some of the roles relinquished by them. While the therapist initially accepted the role of familiar guide in communicating with the hearing world, she paved the way for independent functioning by always stressing their partnership in seeking information and clarification of issues related to Mrs. T and Tommy. A second less acceptable role Mrs. T tried to delegate was that of Tommy's surrogate caretaker. When the therapist firmly refused, Mrs. T's anger and disappointment were evidenced in her facial expression and by her sullen behavior, yet the ground rules were grudgingly accepted. These brief, condensed examples are indications of the delicate balance between gratification, limit-setting, and the encouragement of appropriate autonomous action which formed the backbone of therapeutic work with Mrs. T, and are, of course, a mirror of early maternal functions.

The developing therapeutic relationship was heralded by Mrs. T's growing effort to understand and be understood, to look to the therapist for explanations, and to ask for her if Mrs. T arrived early. Over a period of time Mrs. T began to model some of her behavior on that of the therapist, and eventually indicated at least a minimal awareness of the nursery's potential for contributing to

her own growth and Tommy's, shown in her regular attendance and by her increased willingness to tolerate activities
and behaviors in Tommy previously prohibited.

Primary areas of intervention in our work with
Tommy and his mother as a dyad included attempts to
modify the lack of mutuality in the feeding situation, the
encouragement of a more empathic response to cues, and
the promotion of reciprocal participation in early games
and emerging forms of symbolic play. When this was accomplished, it was primarily through "voicing" Tommy's
unspoken needs for Mrs. T. At the same time, care was
taken to address evocations of her own early experience
elicited by the current relationship to her infant son. For
instance, many of our efforts were aimed at helping Mrs. T
to relax overly restrictive prohibitions regarding Tommy's
play and exploration. Mrs. T's particularly negative response to any kind of messy play seemed related to both
the content of such play and to the issues of autonomy and
control vis-à-vis the child, the nursery, and the therapist.
On his part, even at 11 months, Tommy's ability to control
his impulses was truly remarkable. In one instance, about
to poke his finger in a small dish of water, Tommy looked
at his disapproving mother and withdrew his hand, continuing to stare solemnly at the dish.

These issues, reflecting conflicts of Mrs. T in which
her son had become embroiled, were more easily understood than resolved. Because early development progresses so rapidly, it seemed essential for Tommy to gain
freedom from his mother's undue constriction, which was
jeopardizing the possibility for optimal development. Nevertheless, we were at this point reluctant to intervene directly with Tommy, reasoning that what might appear fa-
cilitative for him might in fact engender confusion and
conflict because of his mother's prohibitions. Equally important, we felt that encouraging Tommy in face of Mrs.
T's proscriptions, might not be tolerable for his mother

and therefore not supportive of their relationship. We were also well aware that allowing Tommy's participation in maternally prohibited activities might threaten this young mother's fragile sense of autonomy in relation to her child and might also undermine our therapeutic relationship by subordinating her needs to those of her son. Interventions instituted from the beginning of treatment seemed to make it possible for Mrs. T to eventually permit some activities previously forbidden. While for many months we honored her prohibitions, we also talked about Tommy's need to explore different materials, pointed out other children's enjoyment of various activities, and voiced Tommy's obvious longing to become involved. Concurrently, we brought to his mother's attention, both Tommy's need for her approval and her part in lifting his inhibitions. Very gradually, Mrs. T began to allow Tommy a broader range of activities that could be drawn on in our work with him without cost to her sense of autonomy, control, and self-esteem.

It is important to note that direct work with Tommy, initiated as his mother became less restrictive, by no means bypassed Mrs. T. Our awareness of her tendency to maintain control of Tommy's activities, along with our clinical judgment that her needs should not be subsumed by Tommy's, insured her inclusion in nursery life during each session. Mrs. T was included by the therapist as participating observer in work with Tommy, and, when tolerable for Mrs. T, as an important contributor to their activities. At the very least, some part of each session was given over to Mrs. T's needs, if only to offer her a favorite snack and catch up on her daily life and concerns.

Although restitutive interventions were, of course, an element of our work with Tommy, treatment dealt with a variety of developmental issues. For example, we felt that the inhibition of aggression might underlie Tommy's subdued and constricted affect and his essentially passive mode of interacting with the environment. Our interventions grew out of a twofold observation. First, Tommy's affect brightened considerably when he engaged in aggressively tinged activities. Second, activities which involved aggressive components seemed to lend energy and drive to Tommy's general level of activity and affect. Early in treatment many channels for the expression of even nonhostile aggression were restricted by Mrs. T's prohibitions and Tommy's inhibitions. Gross motor functions were also greatly inhibited in Tommy but because they were not expressly curtailed by Mrs. T we turned to them as alternate routes of expression, encouraging throwing, banging, and kicking. Toys employed in these activities became objects of interest and gave impetus to exploration. Soon, Tommy's pleasure and interest elicited his mother's participation, marking the inauguration of reciprocal games, with the therapist intervening only to help them sustain their reciprocity or elaborate their play.

Like many parents, Mrs. T thought play was "fun" for Tommy but was unable to consider the developmental implications of most play activities, nor did she sense that play might be an arena for the growth of reciprocity between them. Perhaps because of Mrs. T's own early experience, play with Tommy was neither spontaneous nor afforded her pleasure. Thus, in addition to the dearth of early reciprocal games, neither Tommy nor his mother initiated semisymbolic or symbolic play. For reasons that are not clear, Mrs.T seemed unable to endow objects with anything but their most concrete attributes. Unlike Jeff's mother, she had never played with dolls and dampened Tommy's emerging interest in dolls with her obvious lack of enthusiasm. Both Mrs. T and Tommy seemed to need the therapist to fuel their own interest in pretend play, and perhaps more important, to become caught up in the pleasure of pretending. Probably because they touched on early yearnings in both, pretend games in which Mrs. T and Tommy took turns as the baby who is fed, patted, and put to bed, were especially enjoyed, and played out repeatedly. Gradually Tommy was able to extend these activities to doll play, progressing from discrete behaviors such as lotioning body parts to a more integrated awareness of the whole doll, feeding, bathing, or putting it to sleep. Other instances of deferred imitation, such as playing out his father's interests and vocation were looked for, encouraged, and elaborated. Careful observation of Tommy's activity also became helpful in supporting incipient communications about absent people and events and in encouraging the sharing of experience between Tommy and his mother. For instance, when Tommy was 25 months, he was observed at the mirror punching the air and touching his lip. Brought to his mother's attention, Tommy's behavior was explained by her as a reenactment of a fight with his cousin who hurt Tommy's lip, prompting Mrs. T to sign, gesture, and talk about the incident to Tommy who responded with enthusiastic delight to their first real conversation.

Because Mrs. T was generally unable to help Tommy in the resolution of developmental issues and conflicts, often becoming engaged with him in bitter struggles for control, play became the primary vehicle for mastery. Problems related to toilet training and the process of becoming accustomed to hearing aids, both involving intense struggles between Tommy and his mother, were resolved largely through play. Once offered opportunities, Tommy worked diligently at play around the insertion of ear molds and the fitting of aids. Over the course of treatment this play progressed from mouthing, biting, throwing, and hiding play molds and aids or their surrogates, to a primitive kind of role-play where Tommy, as doctor, aided dolls and therapist. That part of our work which focused on mastering through play essentially passive experiences such as the making of ear mold impressions, was also an

important factor in Tommy's eventual acceptance and excellent use of hearing aids.

By 3, Tommy was exuberant and spontaneous; he
had progressed from a generally passive infant with severe
separation anxiety, constricted affect, and limited motor
activity to a comfortable, expressive, energetic 3-year-old.
For Mrs. T many of the limitations described earlier such
as a tendency toward rigidity, concreteness, and the limited capacity for self-reflection remained. In addition to
increased autonomous functioning, however, we noted a
greater empathy, particularly in relation to her child. For
example, when Tommy's ear molds were initially made for
his hearing aids, Mrs. T anxiously and rigidly held her
distraught son facing away from her. Within a year, she
was spontaneously able to hold him facing her, soothing
him by holding him close, patting him and crooning to
him. We also observed some modulation of her rigidity
along with a growing playfulness in part permitted by her
identification with the therapist. The vignette illustrates
the development of some capacity to regress in the service
of mutuality with her son, within the tripartite structure,
which we think facilitated the regression and its adaptive
modification. When Tommy first showed interest in the
small nursery slide, Mrs. T had to be enticed to sit at the
bottom and catch him. Soon play around the slide became
a favorite pastime for Tommy and his mother. Some
months later, Mrs. T slid down this very small slide, mo-
tioning for Tommy and the therapist to catch her, and as
the nursery year ended, Mrs. T took Tommy in her arms,
climbed to the top of the stairs, and slid down with her
son.

Discussion

As the preceding cases illustrate, the terrible misfor-
tune of giving birth to an organically impaired infant

places innumerable burdens on the adaptive capacities of parents and on the developmental process, as they interweave. For parents, the diagnosis of a child's handicapping condition causes profound suffering, in most cases limiting aspects of individual functioning, and to varying degrees undermining marital and family relationships. Parental responses evoked by the handicap may also limit positive investment in the infant which provides nourishment and structure within and across all developmental lines (Weil, 1978).

Our intervention has the interrelated aims of alleviating parental distress, supporting the parent–child relationship, and facilitating the deaf infant's emerging ego capacities, as reflected in affective and cognitive functioning. We have approached issues related to these concerns within a modified tripartite framework, viewing parent and child as a clinical entity (Greenspan, 1980). The kind of intervention we describe is, of course, one of a number of treatment methods addressing the earliest needs of children. In the following discussion, using deaf infants and their parents as an example, we will explore some of the advantages, disadvantages, and special therapeutic issues relating to this model which we believe has relevance for other parent–child populations at risk for a variety of psychological, socioeconomic, and/or organic causes.

As Fraiberg notes (1980), the birth of an infant may reawaken long quiescent conflicts in parents which have the potential of becoming available to treatment. This may be even more apparent following the birth of a handicapped child. In any case, the actual presence of the baby in treatment can promote the therapeutic process by evoking intense feelings which very quickly become reflected in parent–child interaction. The opportunity to observe such interaction provides the therapist with a rich and ongoing source of insight into the nature and quality of the relationship (Mahler, 1968), especially as it seems to encourage or discourage a growth enhancing environment for the child (Greenspan, 1980). When parent and child are together in treatment, the link between the child's activities and the therapist's observations has an immediacy for parents that might not be possible for a parent seen only individually. The immediacy of treatment can also be therapeutically utilized to gradually sharpen parental understanding and attunement to the baby's cues and needs, and offers access into aspects of the parents' own early experience which is often mirrored in parental behavior toward the child. Differing parental capacities and adaptive styles are naturally to be respected. However, when maladaptive patterns in parent–child interactions arise that seem to affect critical developmental tasks, they can be readily identified and worked with. For example, without the actual presence of both Mrs. T and Tommy, it is doubtful whether the therapist would have had insight into the often subtle interplay between Mrs. T's pervasive prohibitions and the inhibitions that impeded Tommy's exploration of self and surroundings. Nor could she have intervened as effectively in ways that supported both developmental strivings and the relationship among therapist, parent, and child.

When baby and parent are included in treatment, the therapist also frequently becomes a catalyst for playful exchanges that afford the dyad a deep sense of mutual pleasure and satisfaction. Parent and child are helped to appreciate and respond to each other's initiation of play activity through the therapist's active engagement of both, and by her obvious enjoyment of the participants as well as the activity itself. Often, a parent like Mrs. T acquires a sense of playfulness that becomes available to the relationship as a whole and is employed to defuse tense situations and potential conflict. The therapist's initiation and response to the child's play provides the mother with a model for identification as does the therapist's encouragement of the child's creativity in explorative and symbolic play, and his or her efforts at mastery. Similarly, the parent can identify with the therapist's ability to set limits when needed while at the same time facilitating the continuation of a play episode.

As with all therapeutic work, tripartite treatment is a gradual process. We typically work with families for a minimum of one-and-a-half years, and in some instances are able to continue work with parents who later have other deaf children. Although therapeutic work is usually interrupted between the births of successive deaf children, subsequent intervention is enhanced by the previous therapeutic experience.

Regardless of the length of intervention, parents tend to change their conception of treatment during the course of our work with them. In many cases, the initial tendency to view treatment as primarily benefiting their child enables the parents to accept a therapeutic situation which they might initially find too threatening, particularly since they do not view themselves as needing mental health services. Frequently, they nevertheless become actively engaged in the therapeutic process and ultimately consider this process as valuable for themselves as well as for the child. Because intervention lays the groundwork for an often new and different way of thinking about their own experience, at times nursery participation has resulted in parents seeking individual treatment for themselves or another family member. When clinically warranted, tripartite work also allows other family members to be integrated into the treatment process. In two instances, husbands have shared nursery participation with their wives, each bringing their child to one of the two weekly nursery sessions. Although shared participation naturally raises specific issues and problems which must be continually monitored, both families showed improvement in the parents' relationship with each other and their child.

Among the most important issues raised by the tripartite structure are the implications of the relationship between parent and therapist. In contrast to most individual adult therapies, the nursery therapist is also a real object, a factor which colors and alters transferential issues. Fraiberg (1980) addresses this issue and speaks to the fine balance that must be maintained between the therapist as the supportive mother substitute and as the maternal figure in transference. With Fraiberg, we view this as a significant therapeutic concern and as intricately interwoven with all aspects of treatment.

Competitive feelings evoked in the infant and parent as they each seek the therapist's involvement further complicate the therapeutic relationship. Parental envy toward the infant also may be elicited by the therapist's interest and concern for the baby. Here too, a delicate balance must be maintained between the needs of the parent and child, and the issue dealt with by bringing such feelings to parental awareness as part of the treatment process.

Since treatment of handicapped children usually takes place within an agency context and involves multiple services, feelings about the institution and other professionals further affects transference. Close work with colleagues is essential in order to monitor situations that encourage splitting and dilution of the therapeutic process.

Countertransference issues are also complicated by the tripartite nature of treatment. Not only does the therapist react to the parent and child as individuals but to their relationship and the interaction occurring between them. Work with parents thus tends to reevoke issues from the therapist's own early life more acutely than usually occurs in individual work with adults. The therapist's identification with the child's infantile needs, particularly in relation to the parent, is another potential source of difficulty which if not appreciated also can become a major impediment to treatment (Jan Drucker, Ph.D., 1983, personal communication).

Of equal importance, the therapist must be able to tolerate the more primitive aspects of infancy and toddlerhood as well as the toddler's well-known ambivalence, which is embodied in both fondness and attachment, and in possibly disconcerting anger and rejection. The therapist's understanding of developmental issues along with her responses to them, allows her to intervene appropriately with the child, and to explore with parents, their reactions to behavioral manifestations of developmental conflicts and events.

Additionally, the therapist is often pulled between the needs of the parent and child, and is called upon to make moment-to-moment and long-range judgments about the priorities of needs in such a way that excludes neither member of the dyad for any length of time. While the fast-paced developmental process lends a certain urgency to the needs of the child, parental concerns are more than adjunctive, they are fundamental to their child's growth, and indeed, to the continuation of treatment. In our own experience, countertransference responses are more easily resolved when the parent is viewed not as an extension of the child's treatment but as an integral part of the treatment unit.

The nursery setting adds further complexity to therapeutic work. The presence of other parents offers relief from isolation and an opportunity to share experience, but also limits privacy. Although we have found parents often talk freely in the nursery despite the presence of others, the extent to which a lack of privacy hampers therapeutic efforts, is a continuing question. For the child, the nursery offers an arena for social interaction and meaningful engagement of others besides the mother, an important catalyst to self–object differentiation that may not be as available to impaired infants as it is to children who are born organically intact. As noted in Jeff's case, observations of a toddler's growing interest in other children who are also nursery participants, has proved an indicator of the child's degree of differentiation. Periodic, informal visits by siblings and extended family provide a natural and enjoyable way for close relatives to become familiar with our program and more deeply involved with the deaf child.

Conclusion

The proliferation of new approaches to therapeutic work with infants and their families (Greenspan, 1980) suggests that various treatment methods be conceptualized and described with the goal of understanding their most effective aspects and applications. In this paper, we have described the use of the tripartite model of intervention within the context of a nursery setting to address the developmental needs of deaf infants and the emotional needs of their parents. Our experience suggests the efficacy of this model despite the pitfalls and limitations described, and leads us to propose its suitability for early preventive work with infants designated as being at risk for a variety of causes. We believe this approach is particularly suited to psychotherapeutic work with parents who do not initially consider themselves or their infant as needing mental health services, or who may be unusually resistant to and/ or threatened by individual treatment.

As the two cases illustrate, tripartite treatment also appears effective in its ability to meet a range of dyadic needs. In the first case described, the therapeutic approach was largely insight oriented and served as a prelude to individual work. In the second, because the parent was not self-reflective and had less capacity to deal with internal conflict, change was effected primarily through modeling and by identification with the therapist and through supportive, restitutive measures with the mother and child. But even when the capacity for self-awareness is limited, the therapist's understanding of parental history and dynamics, and of psychoanalytic and developmental principles, guides intervention.

Factors involved in the determination of such intervention require careful and continuing assessment of the child's developmental status and of parental capacities and needs. The question of which developmental phases are best served by tripartite intervention is a salient issue, particularly as development becomes more complex and the child is better able to understand language. It should be noted that in the case of deaf infants their disability did, in fact, permit parent–therapist communication about issues that ordinarily might not be addressed in the presence of a child capable of linguistic understanding. As deaf children acquire language, individual treatment of the child and concurrent treatment of the parent might become clinically indicated.

Other considerations include the degree to which parent and child might be unable to express and resolve aspects of aggression in each other's presence, and as development proceeds, the ways in which symbolic representation of the parent can be encouraged and utilized within a tripartite design. Since this capacity appears to facilitate the resolution of issues related to rapprochement and the attainment of object constancy (Mahler et al., 1975), as well as crucial cognitive advances, it might be important to build gradually increasing separations into the tripartite treatment structure. In our nursery, brief separations occurred naturally, but the question of when therapeutic work is most effectively served by the parent's presence or absence remains a significant theoretical and clinical issue resolved in each case by a dynamic understanding of the integrated nature of developmental and dyadic needs. The idea of treatment within a nursery setting must also be addressed within the context of changing developmental and parental needs. Finally, where pathology pervasively limits parental capacities, the primary need may be for individual therapeutic care. Even in these cases, however, tripartite interventions may prove a critical adjunct to individual work with parents; our experience suggests that a tripartite treatment design may be the most effective model for establishing sustained, meaningful communication with and between both members of the dyad.

References

Drucker, J. (1979), The affective context and psychodynamics of first symbolization. In: *Symbolic Functioning in Childhood*, ed. N. R. Smith & M. B. Franklin. Hillside, NJ: Lawrence Erlbaum.

Fields, B. (1979), A theoretical and clinical consideration of libidinal object constancy and object permanence: Issues related to normal development and hearing-impairment. Master's essay. Sarah Lawrence College. Typescript.

Fraiberg, S., ed. (1980), *Clinical Studies in Infant Mental Health*. New York: Basic Books.

Freedman, D. A., Cannady, G., & Robinson, J. S. (1971), Speech and psychic structure: A reconsideration of their relationship. *J. Amer. Psychoanal. Assn.*, 19:765–779.

Galenson, E. (1984), Psychoanalytic approach to psychotic disturbances in very young children: A clinical report. *Hillside J. Psychiat.*, 6/2:221–239.

——— Miller, R., Kaplan, E., & Rothstein, A. (1979), Assessment of development in the deaf child. *J. Amer. Acad. Child Psychiat.*, 18:128–142.

——— Kaplan, E., Miller, R., & Rothstein, A. (1979), The infant nursery project of the Lexington School for the Deaf. In: *Hearing and Hearing Impairment*, ed. L. Bradford & W. Hardy. New York: Grune & Stratton, pp. 429–442.

Greenspan, S. (1980), *Psychopathology and Adaptation in Infancy and Early Childhood: Principles of Clinical Diagnosis and Prevention Intervention*. New York: International Universities Press.

Mahler, M. S. (1968), Infantile psychosis. In: *On Human Symbiosis and the Vicissitudes of Individuation*, Vol. 1. New York: International Universities Press.

——— (1974), Symbiosis and individuation, the psychological birth of the human infant. *The Psychoanalytic Study of the Child*, 29:89–105. New Haven, CT: Yale University Press.

———— (1979), *The Selected Papers of Margaret S. Mahler*, Vol. 1. New York & London: Jason Aronson.

———— Pine, F., & Bergman, A. (1975), *The Psychological Birth of the Human Infant*. New York: Basic Books.

Rainer, J. D. (1976), Some observations of affect, induction and ego development in the deaf. *Internat. Rev. Psychoanal.*, 3:121–128.

Rothstein, A. (1975), Preventive mental health program at the Lexington School for the Deaf. In: *Needs of the Emotionally Disturbed Hearing Impaired Child*, ed. D. Naiman. New York: Deafness Research and Training Center, New York University.

———— (1979), The Mental Health Program at the Lexington School for the Deaf. In: *Hearing and Hearing Impairment*, ed. L. Bradford & W. Hardy. New York: Grune & Stratton.

Solnit, A., & Stark, M. (1961), Mourning and the birth of a defective child. *The Psychoanalytic Study of the Child*, 16:523–537. New York: International Universities Press.

Stern, D. (1974a), Mother and infant at play: The dyadic interaction involving facial, vocal and gaze behaviors. In: *The Effect of the Infant on Its Caretaker*, ed. M. Lewis & L. Rosenblum. New York: John Wiley.

———— (1974b), The goal and structure of mother–infant play. *J. Amer. Acad. Child Psychiat.*, 13:402–421.

Weil, A. M. P. (1978), Maturational variations and genetic-dynamic issues. *J. Amer. Psychoanal. Assn.*, 26/3:461–492.

2

Extending the Intervention Process: A Report of a Distressed Family with a Damaged Newborn and a Vulnerable Preschooler

Peter Blos, Jr., M.D., Douglas Davies, Ph.D., M.S.W.

The dyadic form of the intervention process on behalf of very young children is a development of the past two or three decades. Earlier, the mother or both parents were the focus of therapeutic attention, with the baby considered a passive element in the treatment. As infant research progressed and mental health professionals became increasingly aware of the participatory, rather than solely reactive capacity of infants, they began to include infants as active and essential partners of the treatment. This was so whether the intervention was educative, supportive, and/or psychotherapeutic (Fraiberg, 1980). The concept of attachment provided a theoretical framework within which an attempt was made to facilitate mother–infant communication, understanding, and mutual pleasure (Greenspan and Pollock, 1980). When attachment was difficult or the process was threatened because of the infant's own deficits (e.g., prematurity, congenital or birth deficit),

51

maternal deficiencies (e.g., depression, economic or personal inadequacy, neglectful or abusing impulses), or combinations thereof, the intervention worker or team were necessarily sharply focused on the mother–infant dyad, although, when possible, the father would also be included. The intensity and the demanding nature of this work often precluded attention to other children in the family.

Several times, over recent years, it has been noted that besides the infant upon whom everyone's concern was focused, there was also a young toddler hovering in the background. The parents might make passing disappointed comments about the toddler or complain about some recent bad behavior; but, they were usually too preoccupied to do more, and on home visits we could only make our own observations.

It has been known for a long time that the 1- to 3-year-old whose family expects a new baby invariably experiences many thoughts, fantasies, and ambivalent feelings about this situation. The toddler expresses these reactions through behavior and, if language is available, through words. Under normal circumstances most parents are quite able, perhaps with guidance from the pediatrician, well-baby nurse, or developmental specialist, to help the toddler at such a time and to facilitate appropriate adaptations to this new and developing situation. On the other hand, if tragedy strikes and both family and medical staff are preoccupied with matters pertaining to the survival and possible compromised functioning of a critically ill or damaged newborn, the toddler may silently be placed in high risk. The toddler's essential vulnerability is compounded because the developmental gains most needed for coping with such a situation (e.g., the sense of self as autonomous, the capacity for mental representation of the mothering figure, and language) are recent, and thus not only fragile but also subject to disruption (Mahler, Pine, and Bergman, 1975). Furthermore, the characteristic and normal behavioral expressions of anxiety for the toddler, such as provocative and obnoxious behavior, disruptions of habit training as in toileting, eating, sleeping, as well as clinging and other regressive behaviors, will inevitably grate on the nerves of already tense, anxious, and fatigued parents. It is important to note that the toddler's difficulties may not be expressed immediately. This discontinuity obscures the relationship between cause and effect and leaves the parents baffled and annoyed by their unreasonable child. Under these circumstances the seemingly counterproductive behavior on the part of the toddler readily stimulates in the parents the equally counterproductive reactions of anger, repudiation, isolation, and increased demands on the child. Such a spiral of response and reaction begins all too easily and is all too hard to halt.

The case which follows shows how a toddler, Jimmy, by his phase-specific and age-appropriate behavioral and verbal reactions to threat of maternal loss, reactive anxiety, and extended family stress became, as it were, a lightening rod, drawing upon himself the expression of parental strain, anger, and worry. Jimmy and his mother became caught in such a negative spiral following the birth of a severely damaged baby. Consequently, it became necessary to extend the intervention from mother and baby to a second pair, mother and Jimmy.

In order to best demonstrate such a clinical situation it is necessary to tell the story of the entire intervention. In addition, a follow-up intervention initiated, after two years, by a call from the mother will also be described. This second and briefer contact with the family shows how the initial trauma, with its unconscious components, reverberated like a recurrent bad dream for each member of the family who had been caught in its web.

At the time of Alan Emery's birth, one of us (PB) was engaged in making weekly rounds with the staff on the

Holden Neonatology Intensive Care Unit (NICU) at the University of Michigan Medical Center. The second author (DD) was the parent–infant worker who did the clinical work with the family, using the first author as consultant.

Case Report

INTRODUCTION

Alan had been delivered at a local hospital by emergency caesarean section because of intrauterine fetal distress. He was large for gestational age, a postterm infant (4.9 kg), and had suffered severe birth asphyxia as part of a meconium aspiration syndrome. Apgars had been 1 and 4, his initial heart rate had been 40. Because of his extremely grave condition he had been immediately transferred to the Holden NICU at the University of Michigan Medical Center. At 29 hours of age he had been placed on an Extra Corporal Membrane Oxygenator (ECMO).[1] While on ECMO the baby had developed seizures which required both phenobarbital and dilantin for control. He had also experienced a complete renal shutdown for several hours. After four days and nine hours, he had stabilized sufficiently to be removed from ECMO, although he required hood oxygen for twelve more days. He continued to improve and, on his seventeenth day of life, was transferred to the Moderate Care Neonatal Unit on room air. He remained there for a medically uneventful month until discharge. No seizures had occurred since his removal

Acknowledgments. We would like to acknowledge and thank Dr. Dietrich Roloff, Director of the Holden NICU at the University of Michigan Medical Center, for his supportive interest in the case itself and for reviewing this material.
[1]ECMO is an external form of heart–lung apparatus which is in research development. It is currently only recommended in situations where, without its use, infant death is highly probable.

from ECMO, but he was maintained prophylactically on phenobarbitol.

With the help of skilled care and highly advanced medical technology Alan had made a spectacular recovery. But his mother, who had been told that Alan's birth asphyxia had caused damage to the brain and that he might be mentally retarded, was understandably anxious and agitated. It was notable that her questions, already characterized as ceaseless, now shifted from those focused on survival to issues of long-term prognosis. "*How* retarded?" she asked. "Can he be cared for at home? Will he ever be able to go to school? Will he have to be institutionalized?" Of course, at this time no firm answers could be given and the only answer possible—we'll have to wait and see—was hardly reassuring.

Because of Mrs. Emery's increasing and unrelieved anxiety and agitation a referral to the Infant Psychiatry Unit in the Child Psychiatry Service seemed in order. The NICU staff was especially concerned because the mother seemed so unable to take in the answers to her own incessant and repetitive questions. An added unknown was Mr. Emery, who was in chronic ill-health and perceived by the staff as passive. Would Mrs. Emery's emotional state interfere with her observed capacity to care for this difficult baby?

ASSESSMENT

I (DD) first met with Mr. and Mrs. Emery in the hospital immediately after I had attended a predischarge planning meeting with the multidisciplinary hospital staff. Alan was now 5½ weeks old. Mrs. Emery was a white, 37-year-old mother (Gravida 7, Para 5, AB, 2). Mr. Emery, the father, was black and, as we were later to learn, permanently disabled.

Both parents were stunned by the news that tests had confirmed not only that Alan had sustained brain damage of undetermined extent, but also a severe bilateral hearing loss. Mrs. Emery was clearly anxious as she attempted to sort through the potential meanings of brain damage and deafness for Alan's subsequent development. Mr. Emery was more concerned about how they would be able to follow through on the large number of services the hospital staff had recommended for Alan. I offered to help them organize these recommendations by devising orders of priority for them and also to provide an ongoing assessment of Alan's development. During this first interview, I asked briefly about the family. I learned that the Emerys had two other young children, Jimmy, age 2, and Paul, age 5. Jimmy and Paul had been staying with a family friend for nearly three weeks while Mrs. Emery, still recovering from the caesarean, was preoccupied with Alan's condition. Mrs. Emery's teenage son and daughter from a previous marriage also lived at home and had lived at home throughout these events. I learned that Mr. Emery was permanently disabled by a heart condition and could not expect to return to any work. The family's sole income was his disability benefits. Mrs. Emery referred to her "nerves," and wondered if I could arrange for medication. I said she would need an appointment with a psychiatrist and I would arrange that for her with one at the Infant Psychiatry Program.

Two days later, I met with Mr. and Mrs. Emery as they visited Alan in the moderate care nursery. Because of the medical reports and Mrs. Emery's anxiety, I had prepared myself to see a baby who showed little responsiveness. Alan was a large, placid infant who could focus on his mother's face. He watched her alertly as she smiled and talked to him. The nurses showed the parents how Alan was able to follow a slowly spinning mobile toy with his eyes.

Mrs. Emery began to tell me how much progress Alan had made. He had been comatose at birth, she said, and she had believed he would never wake up. She was holding Alan on her lap as she told me this and she turned to him saying, "Yes, you were lying so still, we thought you'd never wake up. But you did, and look at you now." While Mr. Emery held the baby, she told me the story of his birth. She had known something was wrong the day before because he had stopped moving. She had called her doctor, who had reassured her. But the next day, she was sure something was wrong and went to her hospital emergency room. She said that after being examined, she was taken immediately to the operating room. She was awake during the C-section surgery which was then performed. She realized something was wrong with her baby when she saw the doctors frantically trying to resuscitate him. Later, she would expand the story, adding that she had been convinced the baby was dead, and that the doctors were lying to her when they said he was alive because they wanted to cover up their mistakes. However, just before Alan was urgently transferred to the Holden NICU, a doctor had her feel the baby's chest. She could feel his heart beating.

During this second visit, it was clear that both parents were optimistic about their baby's future. Mrs. Emery was understandably anxious about his coming home, but it was striking how being in physical and affective contact with her baby seemed to calm her.

Following these first two interviews, it was easy to appreciate Mrs. Emery's level of anxiety and agitation in terms of the multiple stresses which she had had to endure. Yet, her attentiveness and appropriate attachment behavior with Alan seemed to bode well. Despite the unclear and troubling prognosis, the parents' optimism at this time about Alan's future was not considered unusual. It was, to be sure, a defensive optimism, but it facilitated psychic consolidation and was a welcome hiatus in a difficult period. The expectation was that it would be transitory, a pause before having to cope with the problems which lay ahead. In addition, it seemed a hopeful sign that the Emerys indicated a receptiveness to my offer to help. Mrs. Emery's request for "nerve medicine" indicated some prior experience with this modality of stress relief, but the details were not requested.

It is frequently difficult to predict the effect of current stress upon a person and a family. It is necessary to underscore that there was little indication at this time of how seriously the stress would affect Mrs. Emery in the days before and after Alan's discharge. Situations have been observed where parental behavior on the neonatal ward was exemplary but proved to be a well-developed facade behind which lay severe personal and family pathology. Conversely, what appeared to the staff as highly idiosyncratic and difficult parent behavior which aroused considerable concern, could turn out to be short lived and not prognostic of severe pathology. One can only conclude that it is important to reassess constantly the parental and family adaptation to stress, both on the ward and after discharge. One must be ever alert to change, whether it be improvement or deterioration.

Only in retrospect was it possible to realize the causes and extent of Mrs. Emery's agitation as the baby's discharge approached, and the effect which her extreme disorganization had upon the professionals responsible for planning and coordinating the baby's care. From the pediatric staff's point of view, Alan was ready for discharge, and it was correctly understood that the Infant Psychiatry Program was working with Mrs. Emery and her infant son. The pediatricians arranged over the weekend to discharge the baby on a Monday. At that time they did not know that Mrs. Emery had already missed an appointment with me, that during the weekend she had been brought to the emergency room by ambulance complaining of chest pains, and that, following an examination by their physicians, she had been cleared medically, given Mellaril, and provided with an appointment with the Adult Psychiatric OPD. On Monday, Alan was discharged as planned, and in the morning the NICU social worker called to inform me of this. Mrs. Emery, as was entirely consistent with her deepening turmoil, neither kept her Monday appointment, called me to tell me of these developments, nor informed the pediatric staff of her visit to the emergency room the night before.

The key to this confusing state of affairs must lie in the different ways Mrs. Emery presented herself to the doctors and staff concerned with Alan, and those concerned with her individually. The pediatric staff, having observed her with Alan many times, saw her as a competent mother who was appropriately anxious about her son's condition. The emergency room staff heard her somatic complaints and correctly perceived them as evidence of anxiety. However, she had not provided them with a link between her symptoms and her baby's condition or imminent discharge. Finally, as described above she had interrupted her contact with me. It must be concluded that unconsciously and defensively Mrs. Emery needed to disrupt professional coordination because of her fears of fantasied consequences. More would be learned about this later.

I reached Mrs. Emery by phone, on Tuesday, the day following Alan's discharge. She said that Alan was doing well, but that she was feeling terrible because she had not been able to sleep for three nights. She again asked me to arrange an appointment with the Infant Psychiatry Program's psychiatrist, which I did. At this point I still did not know, and she did not tell me, about her visit to the emergency room nor of her referral to adult psychiatry. (I am equally certain that those programs did not know at that time of her involvement with us.) When the Infant Program psychiatrist informed me on Wednesday that Mrs. Emery had canceled her appointment, I called her again. This time, she asked me many questions in an agitated and frantic way. She repeatedly tried to establish what my role would be. "Would I talk with her about the baby's development?" "Would I see her alone at my office?" "Wasn't it the job of a psychiatrist to see her if she wanted to talk about her problems?" I assured her that I would try to understand Alan and would monitor his development. She said, "So, you'll be working with the baby, and if I need someone to talk to I can see the psychiatrist." I agreed. It seemed that although she wanted help for herself, she was unable to come in on her own behalf because she was afraid of what might be uncovered. It was easy to suspect that she feared being exposed as somehow responsible for her baby's damage. Because I could sense her increased disorganization and ineffectiveness over the phone, I suggested a home visit that very evening.

When I arrived at 9:00 P.M. Mrs. Emery was lying down. She did not get up. She appeared severely depressed and anxious. She described tremendous headaches and pains all through her body. She had not been sleeping—her husband said she had been up in the middle of the night dusting furniture. She talked in an agitated manner, and, at times, her thinking became tangential with some loosening of associations. She showed me letters from her sister and mother, which she said were depressing. She felt there were obscure references to death in the letters. "What was her mother trying to do to her by talking about death?" "How could they write such letters at a time like this? Were they trying to drive her crazy?" Again, she told the story of the caesarean, focusing on how she had thought the baby was dead. I said I thought she was tremendously upset by what had happened to her and her baby, and that she was worried about her baby. She agreed and again asked for medication. Because of the psychotic features in her presentation, I suggested an adult psychiatric evaluation this time so that she would be sure to get the care she needed and to separate this more clearly from the Infant Psychiatry Program. She accepted. When she went to the Adult Psychiatric Clinic the next day, Thursday, she was able to pull herself together and appeared only very anxious, not psychotic. However, when I came for the next home visit one day later, Mrs. Emery was clearly psychotic. She had constructed a paranoid delusional system involving the assumption that the adult clinic psychiatrists and other doctors wanted to drive her crazy, so she'd have to be hospitalized. The doctors were monitoring her movements and were taking pictures of her, so that everyone would know who she was. She felt she was a guineapig for the doctors and the hospital, as was Alan. The psychosis, with the persecutory delusions, the externalization of blame, and the fantasies that she was being experimented upon and damaged, was understood as a desperate defense against the overwhelming guilt that she had damaged her baby and the probably unacceptable fury at her doctor who had initially not taken her apprehensions seriously. It seemed clear that the acute psychosis had been precipitated by Alan's discharge, which placed him in her care.

Mrs. Emery was seen for a second interview at the Adult Psychiatric Clinic seven days after Alan had been discharged. It is noteworthy that the interviewing psychiatrist observed that Mrs. Emery, who had brought Alan with her, "Cared well for the baby, feeding and cuddling him appropriately during the interview," despite her obvious persecutory and physical delusions.[2] Hospitalization was recommended, but Mrs. Emery refused, saying she would not allow them to take her away from her baby. The

---

[2]We thank Dr. Susan Theut for sharing her observations.

dosage of Mellaril was increased and an appointment three days hence was given. The day before the appointment, she called and canceled the appointment for delusional reasons.

This was now an acute and difficult situation. Alan had been home for a week, and Mrs. Emery was acutely psychotic. She refused either to take medication or to be hospitalized. Her inner state of mental chaos was reflected in the chaos and anxiety she created in the various personnel and departments of the hospital. Despite this, two home visits during the following week enabled me to observe that although she was manifestly psychotic, Mrs. Emery was quite in touch with her baby. She was responsive to his signs, and able to hold and feed him. Alan took the bottle well, and his bodily needs seemed well attended to. He appeared to be appropriately responsive to his mother. She was also able to speak for Alan, telling her husband to change his diaper or her teenage son to quiet the younger children while he was sleeping. These periods of warm and concerned interaction with Alan alternated with delusional outbursts against the doctors. It appeared that even though Mrs. Emery was psychotic, Alan was not being drawn into her delusional system. On the contrary, her relationship with him was an island of reality for her. Alan also seemed to be thriving.

In concluding the discussion of his tumultuous assessment and emergency treatment period, it must be added that Mr. Emery was very competent in taking care of the baby and his wife, and appeared supportive of his wife. He seemed to agree with her accusations and her delusions which at least kept the couple together. In addition, a public health nurse had been making independent home visits and was monitoring the baby's physical progress, as well as the caretaking he was receiving. Her impressions agreed with mine that Alan was receiving adequate care and that Mrs. Emery was highly invested in him. It was very helpful to have another professional provide independent confirmation of a case that was so difficult and anxiety-provoking. We decided that a home-based, supportive, concretely oriented treatment built upon Mrs. Emery's strengths as a mother would be appropriate. It was noted that she implicitly utilized Alan as an organizer of her experience and the treatment would aim to support her in this. At the same time the public health nurse, the pediatric clinic, and I would closely observe Alan for any indications that he was not being cared for properly at home.

It has been found that babies can serve very well as indicators of the care they are receiving. This is particularly true if one uses the affective indicators of gaze patterns, responsivity, and initiating behavior, as well as the better known physical ones of physical growth and bodily care. In this particular case, it was also felt to be vital not to disrupt the developing maternal and paternal infant attachment process. A strong parental cathexis of this damaged baby was going to be essential for his optimal development. At the same time, we needed to be alert to possible dangers for Alan, and be ready to intervene more actively if necessary.

INTERVENTION: ON THE BABY'S BEHALF

In response to her panic when Alan came home, Mrs. Emery had tried to do everything—clean the house, cook for the family, and take care of the baby. In addition, Jimmy and Paul, the two younger children, had returned home a few days before the baby's discharge and were having their own reactions to the family crisis, especially to the prolonged separation from their mother. They, too, were looking to mother to fulfill their needs. Her husband and adolescent children were trying to stop her from exhausting herself by taking over the household, but Mrs.

Emery experienced this as a criticism, and further evidence of her inadequacy. I suggested that she could not expect to do all she usually did because she was still recovering from major surgery; furthermore, she had been through a very emotionally tiring and painful experience that would make anyone feel drained and overwhelmed. She replied that she was afraid the house would turn into a shambles. Mr. Emery firmly said he would not allow this to happen. I added that everything might not be up to her standards, but that I could see that her husband would make sure that the essentials got done. It was, I went on, expecting too much of herself to take care of everything the first week her baby came home from the hospital. Finally, I reminded her, the situation was only temporary, and as she felt better physically, she could return to her accustomed role and tasks. It would be a gradual process and in the meantime, she should concentrate on what was important—taking care of Alan, and resting to allow her body to recover. During this emergency period following Alan's discharge, I made home visits twice weekly for two weeks and then shifted to once weekly visits as Mrs. Emery's anxiety and delusions began to lessen and as the family settled into a routine that included Alan.

By the end of one month, there were only occasional flashes of the psychotic symptoms. As Mrs. Emery invested more and more in Alan, she became increasingly oriented to reality. The therapeutic work during this period focused on a weekly assessment of Alan's development. At each weekly home visit, Mrs. Emery, who was an astute observer, would report her observations about Alan's behavior and raise questions about its meanings. For instance, she had noticed that his left eyelid drooped slightly; was this the result of the seizures after birth? She was convinced that he responded to sounds by turning his head; could the diagnosis of severe hearing loss be inaccurate? We watched Alan together and spoke of our observations. To many of Mrs. Emery's questions, the answer could only be that it was too early to tell how Alan would develop. So far, however, it was obvious that Alan was developing within normal limits affectively and socially. At 2½ months, he was smiling, responding with pleasure when he was cuddled, and crying when he was uncomfortable. To Mrs. Emery, who already had four babies, these were convincing and heartening signs that Alan, in spite of his terrible history, was a normal baby in many ways. Together we noted small steps in development and, less frequently, possible difficulties or delays. Gradually, we were putting together a picture of Alan, which included his strengths and limitations. Soon, Mrs. Emery began introducing me to visiting friends as "the baby's therapist."

Mrs. Emery had noticed early on that Alan was not physically as active as she would have expected and that he tended to keep his right hand clenched. I had agreed with this observation and added that it would be important to ask Alan's doctors about this. After Alan had been home for six weeks (now age 13 weeks), the doctors gave a name to what she had observed—cerebral palsy. The parents were shocked by this diagnosis since they felt Alan had been making such good progress. They had begun to hope that he would eventually catch up and show normal development. Mrs. Emery's psychotic symptoms returned briefly, although in a milder form. She also asked more questions about the long-term effects of cerebral palsy. "Would Alan ever walk?" "Would he lack control of his muscles like another child she had seen?" But, as had been true earlier the answers could not be taken in. They did not help, and neither parent could believe that Alan's cerebral palsy was severe.

Mrs. Emery's unacknowledged sense of responsibility for the damage to her baby, as well as her generally caring nature, led her to make very active efforts to minimize the impact of Alan's physical problems on his future development. The parents wanted to make sure that he got good care immediately. They attempted to get social security disability benefits for Alan, to enroll him in an early intervention program, and to get him a hearing aid through the Crippled Children's Fund. There were many forms to fill out, many phone calls to make, and the process was exhausting and frustrating. I responded with interventions centered around problem solving in support of their pursuit of services for Alan. I listened as they complained about bureaucratic hostility and aloofness and empathized with their difficulties. But I then asserted that we had to keep trying so that Alan would get the services he needed and to which he was entitled. Implicitly, I supported their anger and complaining because it clearly mobilized them to set goals for Alan's care and because Mrs. Emery could adaptively use such concrete problem solving in the service of reorganizing herself. I also made phone calls and wrote letters to agencies and referred them as well to a local organization which did advocacy work on behalf of children with birth defects.

During this period, the work could proceed because I had been able to form an alliance with Mrs. Emery and the family on behalf of her baby. The interventions were aimed at supporting in concrete ways the process of Alan's becoming real for her. I responded to what was potentially adaptive and realistic in her perceptions of Alan rather than responding to the delusional aspects of her thinking. For example, I agreed that it was best for her to be with her baby, without joining in her condemnation of the psychiatrist who, she felt, wanted to take her away from her baby. Earlier, she had made a clear split between "her baby's therapist" and those who wanted to "dig into her mind and drive her crazy." The therapeutic alliance with the positive side of this splitting permitted her to think of me as someone who was helping Alan, not someone who perceived her as having problems which needed help. It was important to respect this defensive splitting since Mrs.

Emery's intense and irrational guilt and blame for what had happened to her baby probably lay behind it, as well as her intense ambivalence about the medical profession. For related reasons, any interpretive work on Mrs. Emery's own thoughts, fantasies, delusions, and emotions, or questions about her past history and experiences had to be avoided. To focus on her own difficulties would, it was believed, only risk a resurgence of the affects and fantasies which had precipitated her psychotic episode. She could only cope with the severe injury to her self-esteem and narcissism and her powerful emotional reactions by psychotic thinking and somatic delusions. It could be determined later whether her ego could or would need to explore this area. Therefore, I quickly accepted that surgery and worry were the cause of her physical symptoms, and that rest and talking would gradually find her feeling physically better.

INTERVENTION: ON THE TODDLER'S BEHALF

So far the story and the work it reports have been devoted to assisting an emotionally precarious mother with a neurologically damaged baby. The psychological emergency had to be dealt with immediately; a mother and baby who could not wait. As the treatment plan slowly took effect all concerned could feel reassured, which allowed me gradually to become aware of Jimmy and Paul, Alan's two young brothers. I began to note the effect which these emotion-laden and dramatic weeks had had upon them and the expression of their reactions. When I first tentatively commented upon these reactions little could be done. Mrs. Emery would recount the bad things Jimmy had done and comment on how mean he was, but she had no capacity to perceive his behavior as having anything to do with the preceding events.

It will be recalled that Jimmy and Paul lived with a friend of the family for nearly a month following Alan's sudden and traumatic birth. They returned home just a few days before Alan arrived. Jimmy was then 25 months old and Paul 5 years of age. Jimmy's reactions to the sudden and prolonged separation were not unusual for a 2-year-old who had previously been securely attached to his mother. But his difficulties were intensified by the fact that his mother was different now. She was preoccupied with the new baby and had turned over his care completely to his father. She would frequently yell at him to go to his room and play and caustically asked when he was going to be a big boy and stop wearing diapers. Mrs. Emery had little tolerance for Jimmy's neediness, which at first was expressed by his refusal to let her out of his sight, and then by his constant requests for food.

Jimmy responded to his mother's apparent abandonment, rejection of him, demandingness, punitiveness, and her agitation with actions that, on the one side, were attachment seeking to calm his anxiety and, on the other side, expressive of his outrage at being treated this way. Although these conflicting and ambivalent feelings were expressed in modes characteristic of a 2-year-old, it was difficult for the parents to see them as intending to elicit his mother's concern and communicate his hurt. He once went to her room and smeared his face with her cosmetics. He was very negative and would have a tantrum if his mother or father refused to give him candy. He broke dishes and unplugged the refrigerator. He gave up his previously partially established bowel training.

Paul, the 5-year-old, dealt with his own pain at mother's unavailability by trying to be a "good boy." Part of this involved manipulating Jimmy to execute the expression of Paul's resentment in some action and then telling on him to gain approval. In an unfortunate combination, Jimmy's natural 2-year-old oppositionalism, his serious anxiety, and his brother's exploitation led his parents to see Paul as "good" and Jimmy as "bad" and "mean." He was quickly becoming a scapegoat in a family that used externalization of hostility and splitting others into good and bad objects as a way to maintain familial and internal psychological stability. It also appeared that Jimmy's behavior represented for Mrs. Emery an acting out of the "craziness" she was trying so hard to suppress in herself.

Jimmy was clearly in considerable difficulty and at psychological risk, yet intervening on his behalf proved difficult. My comments about the impact of the separation and family stress upon the boys were to no avail. Oddly, it was the parents' request for concrete help in disciplining Jimmy, which provided a viable alternative pathway.

I had discovered that Mrs. Emery was most receptive when I talked about Jimmy in terms of normal 2-year-old development. It was easier, for example, for her to hear that many children are not ready for toilet training until they are 2½, than to hear that his recent refusal to use the toilet was reactive to the crisis in the family. I said that 2 was a difficult age and that tantrums, fighting over toys, and resistance to parents were common. The parents spontaneously recalled that Paul had "gotten into a lot of trouble" when he was 2, which indicated and underscored the normality of the behavior and was an improvement from seeing Jimmy as congenitally bad.

Here we see again how sensitive Mrs. Emery was to any hint that there was trouble. Ordinarily, in the case of reactive disturbances during the second and third years of life one attempts to help parents see the child's frustrating behavior as reactive to stress, a combination of fear and anger, so that they will be able to offer reassurance, support, and understanding. Gradually then, the relationship is restored to equilibrium, and the child can move forward again. But, Jimmy's mother could not tolerate the idea that he was vulnerable, had been hurt, and needed her. This awareness only served to stimulate her potent and disruptive feelings of fault, guilt, and blame. In addition, she was recovering from a psychotic episode. Her concrete thinking prevented her from making the causal links between the earlier separation and Jimmy's current overtly angry, provocative, and hostile behavior. Since neither parent was able to look at the causes of Jimmy's behavior, I began talking to him directly. At some point during each home visit—usually on the sidewalk as I was leaving—I would find a chance to talk to Jimmy alone. He was usually there and seemed interested. Jimmy would listen with good attention, but it was difficult to gauge his responses. He would often repeat fragments of what I said in the manner of a 2-year-old who is in a period of rapid language learning. I tried to take advantage of this developmental process by repeatedly putting his experience into simple words. The aim was to provide him with some verbal organization of what had happened. I hoped he could gain some distance from the traumatic events if he could objectify them a bit in language. Over many weeks, I spoke of how worried and scared he had been when his mother had suddenly gone away. I said that his mother had not wanted to leave, but that she needed to because Alan had been very sick. I assured Jimmy that his mother had not left because he had been bad. His mother was home to stay now, and they could all feel better.

When Alan reached 4 to 5 months of age and Mrs. Emery could begin to feel some confidence that he would develop, she could begin to reassure Jimmy herself, as if perceiving Alan as basically safe allowed her to regain a fuller range of affect, be less anxious and depressed, and be more affectively available to her other children. For example, she spontaneously began to reconstruct with Jimmy his experience during the separation. On one occasion, she went with Jimmy and Paul on a visit to the friend with whom they had stayed during the crisis. When Jimmy first saw the house he refused to get out of the car. When asked why by his mother, already an indicator of her returning sensitivity, he told her fearfully that he did not want to stay there. Mrs. Emery now could see he was frightened and understood that he did not want to be separated from her again. When she told me about this incident she said, "When I saw how scared he was, I knew he must have had a hard time there. It was all a big mess. He didn't know where I was and what was going on."

Mrs. Emery now could understand that Jimmy had suffered during his separation from her, an idea she had rejected when I had suggested it earlier. We could begin to reinterpret Jimmy's difficult behaviors as reactive to the separation from his mother. On her own initiative, Mrs. Emery asked her friend what Jimmy had been like when she was in the hospital and learned that he had been very quiet and withdrawn. "When I heard that," she said to me, "I knew he'd had a hard time because he was never like that. He was always full of energy." I said that he must have missed her a great deal because 2-year-olds normally have great trouble tolerating long separations from their mothers. I added that it was common for 2-year-olds to get into a lot of behavioral difficulty after a separation. I suggested, too, that Paul had been upset by the separation and that he had used Jimmy's troublesome behaviors as a means of trying to win her favor. As Mr. and Mrs. Emery began to notice that Paul sometimes attempted to get Jimmy into trouble, they became less punitive.

My weekly home visits continued until Alan was 9 months of age. During the fifth, sixth, and seventh months of life he made steady, if slow, gains cognitively and affectively and was clearly attached to his mother as she was to him. His hearing had improved, and the auditory damage now appeared minimal. He was such a responsive and active baby that it was easy to have one's concerns about severe mental retardation allayed. Due to the cerebral palsy he continued to demonstrate slow motor development. However, a Bayley administered when he was 7 months old showed he had lagged two months behind on *both* the mental and motor scales. At 7½ months of age, his head circumference was below the fifth percentile (42 cm), while his height was in the 75th percentile (72.5 cm), and his weight was in the 25th percentile (8 kg).

Despite these ominous signs of developmental delay and brain damage, it was striking during my visits after Alan was 7 months old, how Mrs. Emery had finally been able to form a coherent picture of him. It appeared that she assimilated in some way that his development would be steady, though slow. Many questions remained, but she asked them less stridently, because she knew that Alan was not the damaged, lifeless baby she had first seen. She had also developed a confidence that he would continue to surprise the doctors and herself with his progress.

I noticed that she was warming up to Jimmy and encouragingly talking about the big boy things he could do. She could even laugh at some of his antics which had angered her just a few months before. He had been taken out of the scapegoat role, even though he continued to be oppositional.

INTERVENTION: TERMINATION

Mrs. Emery's stable remission from the acute psychosis, the observed stability in the mother–infant relationship, and her renewed ability to parent Jimmy and Paul more empathically provided me with a basis to initiate termination. Aware that Jimmy and Paul had not worked through their responses to the family crisis, I suggested that further treatment could be helpful to them. Mr. and Mrs. Emery refused this offer. They felt that Jimmy's behavior had improved a great deal and did not seem to appreciate that he might still be internally troubled. Within this context, Mrs. Emery spontaneously retold the story of Alan's birth and hospitalization in even greater detail than had been possible earlier. For instance, she now recovered memories of her fear during the caesarean section. For the first time, she described to me how terrible Alan had looked when she first saw him: "He was still hooked up to the machine [ECMO]. He was so pale and lying so still that he looked almost dead." While she remembered how upset and frantic she had been, she did not show any awareness of having been psychotic about Alan's damaged condition nor did she express any guilt or anger.

During the month-long termination process, I continued to describe to Mrs. Emery Jimmy's and Paul's reactions to their separation from her. Finally, I was able to link their difficult behavior following Alan's discharge with her own upset. Since Jimmy and Paul were present during these meetings, the termination process gave the boys a fuller opportunity to understand the traumatic events.

FOLLOW-UP

One-and-one-half years after termination Mrs. Emery called me. Alan was now 2 years and 4 months of age, Jimmy was 4, and Paul was 7. She first said she had wanted to let me know how well Alan was doing and described proudly how the baby the doctors said would not walk until he was 5 had begun walking a month ago. Only much later in our conversation did she mention that she was concerned about Jimmy. She told me that he was once again very defiant and getting into trouble at home. A few months before, following an incident when she had been very angry with him, he had stuck a live wire from the stereo in his mouth. He had sustained a transient seizure and a serious electrical burn at the edge of his mouth (1.5 cm). He had been hospitalized overnight for observation, but there had been no complications. I offered to make a home visit four days later, and she accepted. When I arrived no one was home, and a neighbor told me that Mrs. Emery was in the hospital for surgery. She had not mentioned surgery in her call to me, and I was puzzled. I called the home the next day and found out that Mrs. Emery had not yet gone to the hospital but was scheduled for a hysterectomy in the next few days. I would not be able to schedule a home visit until after she had returned from the hospital.

This ambivalent beginning strongly suggested that Mrs. Emery's call had been prompted by unconscious fears of a repetition of the earlier traumatic hospitalization, surgery, and family crisis when Alan was born. On the telephone she sounded characteristically enthusiastic and forceful but without undue anxiety, agitation, or psychotic thinking. Characteristically, Jimmy had again been placed in the scapegoat role. Nevertheless, Mrs. Emery clearly knew whom to call when a particular stress (gynecological surgery and hospitalization) confronted the family. Her doing so provided me with an opportunity to help the family work through a little bit more of the earlier severe trauma, as well as giving us an occasion for a follow-up assessment. In sum, the follow-up visits became a brief intervention focusing on the family's current reaction to Mrs. Emery's brief hospitalization and separation. Jimmy and Paul, who had been rendered extremely vulnerable by the traumatic experiences surrounding Alan's birth, would now be my primary concern. I recognized that because the reawakened affective reactions to the earlier trauma were being acted out rather than being remembered, repetition rather than mastery would take place. Thus, my principal task would be to attempt to build memory bridges between the traumatic events of two-and-a-half years ago and the present stimulus situation.

At the beginning of the first visit Mrs. Emery briefly described her uncomplicated five-day hospitalization. Then she launched into an angry account of Jimmy's behavior. She was particularly upset because he had emptied out some inhalers containing her asthma medication. She also said that a neighbor had caught him putting bricks under the tires of her car and she thought he had intended to wreck the tires. While Jimmy, who was cast once again in the bad boy role, was surly and very anxious, Paul, who also looked somewhat anxious and withdrawn, was presented as the good boy who had told on Jimmy. I suggested that Jimmy was reacting once again to a separation from his mother and the heightened family anxiety. I reviewed how frightened and upset he had been when Alan was born and his mother had of necessity been gone so long. There was also the long crisis when she had been so worried about Alan. I said that I knew that even though this time it had been neither a traumatic hospitalization nor an emergency, Mrs. Emery had been anxious before the surgery. I suggested that Jimmy and Paul had known she was worried too, and that both children had probably feared a repetition of the events surrounding Alan's birth. Evidence for this was that they were both behaving as they had then. Once again, Jimmy was getting into trouble and Paul was being good and telling on Jimmy.

The following week when I arrived Mrs. Emery reported that she had caught Paul in the act of emptying an inhaler. When she realized that he had been doing at least some of the mischief for which Jimmy had been blamed, she had spoken with her neighbor and learned that *both* boys had been involved in putting bricks under the tires. With Paul and Jimmy present as we spoke, I suggested that throwing away the medicine probably had a special meaning: medicine was associated with her sickness, hospitalization, and separation. By throwing the medicine away they were denying that their mother could become sick and go to the hospital again. At this point she began to understand what her children had expressed behaviorally. She said, "Yes, and when they put the bricks under the tires it was just before I was going to the hospital. They didn't want me to go." I said to the children, "I understand why you wanted to get rid of the medicine and put the bricks under the tires. You never want mom to go to the hospital again. You remembered how scary it was for you when mom went to the hospital when Alan was born and you were scared that it would be like that again."

Because the dynamics of this minor crisis recapitulated those of the period after Alan's birth, the intervention was a brief version of the previous extended one. While it offered Mr. and Mrs. Emery, Jimmy, and Paul another opportunity to clarify their past experience, neither boy has been able to sufficiently work through the earlier trauma, and I felt that each remained particularly vulnerable to future separations. Although Mr. and Mrs. Emery gained some understanding of the impact of the previous crisis on the children, Mrs. Emery, when she is under duress, continues to read her children's behaviors at face value rather than perceiving them as reactions to stress or requests for help and reassurance. Treatment was again offered for the boys but again refused. The occasion of this renewed contact did permit me to observe Alan, the originally identified patient, and to review his pediatric records. We assume the reader will be as curious about Alan as we were. A brief summary of my report at the time of the second intervention follows.

At two-and-a-half (30 months) Alan appeared to be moderately retarded. He was microcephalic (below the 5th percentile at 26½ months—45 cm), had cerebral palsy, chronic lung disease, and asthma. Two Bayleys administered at nineteen-and-a-half and twenty-eight months indicated that he was severely delayed (7–10 months) in cognitive development, especially in expressive and receptive language. His motor development was quite delayed (15 months), largely because of the cerebral palsy which affects both legs and arms, the right more than the left. But, he was noted to be animated, social, and clearly attached to his mother. The parents saw continuous if slow developmental progress in all areas and this allowed them to remain optimistic about his development while at the same time recognizing his limitations. So far he has gone far beyond the predictions which the doctors made during the first few months of his life. Alan, much to the doctors' surprise, began walking at 20 months. He is a social, warm, related, and demonstrative child whose parents remain highly invested in him. They have worked hard to provide him with good medical and rehabilitative care and have enrolled him in an early intervention educational program. It is noteworthy that he did not have a strong separation reaction to his mother's five-day absence.

Discussion

The intervention which we have reported began as infant focused. Mrs. Emery has made her needs clearly known through her words and behavior and managed to convey to everyone her intense panic, underlying worry, and desperate need for help. Clearly, she needed immediate assistance if she was going to be able to take care of her badly damaged baby. Alan, in turn, was going to need all the care, receptiveness, and responsivity his parents could muster in order to develop to the best that his damaged neurological system would allow. Neither could wait. The touchstone for a working alliance, as is so often the case, proved to be the mother's intense interest and concern for her baby's well-being.

Jimmy, the toddler, only came to our attention because of our facility's capability to permit home-based treatment. It is doubtful that specific help for Jimmy would have been sought since his "bad" and "mean" behavior was perceived as constitutionally given. In fact, Mrs. Emery and her husband could not consider the possibility that Jimmy's behavior was reactive and therefore treatable. They were already severely overburdened with obvious concerns and uncertainties.

We have reported how Mrs. Emery used splitting as a defense and how this permitted her to utilize the pediatricians and the infant–parent worker on behalf of Alan while perceiving the psychiatrists and other doctors as wanting to harm her. To our surprise, Jimmy, in the same way, became the split-off and projected bad object at home, while other family members were perceived as helpful. There may be historical reasons of which we are unaware why Jimmy was selected as the "bad" and "mean" object. But, unquestionably, his phase specific behavior was an important ingredient in determining this choice.

The worker's concern was aroused by reports of Jimmy's "badness" as well as by knowledge of how vulnerable 2-year-olds are to separations. But he could only observe Jimmy on home visits and bide his time until the parents could begin to hear Jimmy's needs. One must consider that the Alan-centered work, vital in itself, also served to help Mrs. Emery reintegrate, and thereby finally become available to Jimmy. The sequential nature of these two interventions proved to be parsimonious, necessary, and efficient. After five months, the Emerys signaled their readiness to think about Jimmy by raising the problem of his discipline. From this point onward the Alan work and the Jimmy work could proceed simultaneously.

Jimmy's reactions to the sudden, stressful, and disorganizing events which took place in his family are quite typical for a 2-year-old. His stay at the friend's home with his brother was much longer than anyone had anticipated. The emotional shock and the reactive depression he experienced at this sudden and prolonged separation were reflected in the observed change in his demeanor: from an active, lively boy he became a somber, quiet one. Fortunately, there were a few mitigating circumstances such as his brother Paul being with him and the fact that the friend and her home were familiar. Because he was 2, little had been said directly to Jimmy about what was happening, and he had to garner what he could by overhearing others. Often, in situations like Jimmy's, toddlers are seen by adults as being too little to understand what is happening, and it is thereby hoped that the young child can be spared the unpleasant suffering, the emotional pain, and the stressful confusion experienced by the adults. We do not mean to suggest that 2-year-olds like Jimmy can understand the complex events which are taking place around them. But, we think toddlers can grasp simple and direct words which speak about the facts (e.g., the baby is sick, mommy is busy but she will be back), and the emotions (e.g., missing someone, sadness, being mad, worry) which may trouble the toddler. They should be said directly to him and be repeated as the repetition in stories which toddlers love so much. Sometimes improvised stories which incorporate the essential events and probable feelings can be told and retold. The purpose, as we stated earlier when the worker spoke directly and regularly to Jimmy, is to provide naming as a pathway for objectification and recall, to provide alternative concepts for the age-appropriate, egocentric perceptions of causality, and to provide an empathic emotional context of attention. Under the circumstances of our case, the worker's attention was an emergency-based holding action and could not be corrective by itself. It was an attempt to help Jimmy until his mother could be again available to him in a more familiar and understanding way.

Jimmy's behavior on first returning home was not unusual—to follow his mother everywhere and not to let her out of his sight. In his need for reassurance that mother was there and would continue to be there, he tried to stick closely to her. We can readily see that this clinging, regressive behavior expressed his fervent wish not to lose her again. But, at the same time it had the effect upon his mother, as everyone knows who has been exposed to a toddler in such distress, of a silent reproach. If the toddler's expressed hostility and the parents' guilt can be tolerated, then parents can provide affective support through action and words which will slowly help the toddler regain a former level of confident individuation (Mahler, Pine, and Bergman, 1975). Mrs. Emery was psychically unable to do this and reacted to Jimmy as to one who was causing her additional pain. She yelled at him in angry exasperation to go to his room and leave her alone, to grow up, and, essentially, demanded he no longer be dependent on her. Thus, Jimmy did obtain his mother's attention, but not in the positive, reassuring way he or we might have wished. For toddlers who are reacting to significant object loss, any attention is better than being ignored and feeling totally abandoned.

The regression and misbehavior escalated. His partial toilet training was lost. He nagged for food. He smeared his face with his mother's cosmetics, unplugged the refrigerator, broke dishes, and had temper outbursts when he could not have his way. Such behavior is frequently perceived by adults, as it was by the Emerys, as manipulative and "bad" (read hostile). But the usual reaction of not giving in, getting angry, or banishing the toddler turns out to perpetuate the very behavior it is meant to stop. The matter, now muddled, turns into a battle in which everyone loses. To accede to a toddler who is "just trying to get attention" would, it is often feared, reward and reinforce the intolerable behavior. But the absence of response only makes the child more frantic in his provocations. It was at this point that the Emerys asked for help with disciplining Jimmy. This signaled to the worker that they had the mental energy to notice him and to be concerned.

We can profitably look at Jimmy's behavior in three interlocking ways which, in turn, provide us with a rationale for interventive strategies. Our aim was to assist Jimmy and his mother in gaining a rapprochement which would permit appropriate psychic development to take place again. Psychodynamically, Jimmy's behavior expressed his fear of loss, his desperate need for reassurance, his fury at his perceived rejection and abandonment, and his egocentric sense of causing what had happened. Since we were not permitted to treat Jimmy in psychotherapy we do not have confirmatory data for the following hypothesis about what, symbolically, was going on within Jimmy and between him and his mother. However, psychoanalytic theory and clinical work with other mother–toddler pairs suggest that Jimmy's activities during this time were far from random. His clinging behavior and incessant desire for food not only suggest a need for psychic food and nurturance but also a little boy for whom behavior is a language. Applying his mother's cosmetics to his face is a poignant statement if one hears it rightly, as an attempt to be like the mother—close as skin is close and with the same nice mommy smells. Of course it also contains the retaliatory wish to make a mess of, and with, something of value to her. The predictable result of these and other acts—unplugging the refrigerator, breaking dishes—was a "swat" or spanking. Perhaps one can best think of these acts as perverse (i.e., distorted) attachment-seeking behavior which provide some momentary reassurance. But repetition rather than appropriate psychic development is the end result.

Behavioral psychology would describe these acts as provoking punishment—a form of attention, albeit undesirable—which in turn stimulates further "bad" or "mean" behavior. There follows, then, a mutual reinforcement of unwanted behavior on the part of the toddler and parent.

To interrupt this cycle requires rewarding desired behavior with attention of a positive valence and letting the bad behavior extinguish by removing the reinforcement of attention.

A developmental approach to Jimmy's cognitive and psychological abilities and needs provides us with a normative standard. It also helps us anticipate problem areas, common misconceptions, and expectable mental capabilities which can guide us in our intervention. As a body of data it is nonjudgmental and thus often can provide a nonthreatening point of entry for work with parents. This was certainly the case for Mrs. Emery. When she could perceive Jimmy's refusal to get out of the car on a visit to the friend's house as an age-appropriate expression of anxiety rather than stubbornness and ask Jimmy what the trouble was, they were back in communication again.

These three ways of understanding the problem of Jimmy and his mother—the psychodynamic, the behavioral, and the developmental—gave the worker a broad armamentarium from which to choose his initial approach. For Mrs. Emery, an educative and supportive approach based on developmental expectations proved eminently workable and, in time, permitted the behavioral and psychodynamic elements to unfold. The brief second intervention, which focused on Jimmy and Paul, was quickly able to focus on the psychodynamic content of the behavior by recalling similar events of two years ago. Parental understanding thus facilitated better behavioral management—less punishment and more acknowledgment of anxiety (fear of a repetition of the earlier trauma), and more positive reinforcement.

We do believe that these interventions have been helpful and, from a preventive pediatric, developmental, and psychic stance, extremely useful. Alan's social responsiveness and relatedness at 2½ years of age, and the extent of his cognitive and motor development, is, we believe, due in large measure to the good mothering and fathering he has received. He is, of course, badly damaged neurologically; we tend to agree with his parents, however, that he will continue to surprise us in his future development. But, significant problems remain for Jimmy and Paul. Jimmy's "accident" with the live stereo wire was, we think, overdetermined and indicative of psychological difficulties. Paul's penchant for using others to express his hostility and his need to be perceived as a "good" boy also indicate probable troubles for him. It was unfortunate that we were not permitted to work with these boys in a psychotherapy that might have helped them overcome some of the internalized reactions to these traumatic events.

Conclusion

In this report we have shown how intervention on behalf of a vulnerable and neurologically damaged infant could be extended to provide help for a toddler sibling who had been affected by precipitous and prolonged separation from his mother, family, and home. Intervention technique has been discussed, and its conceptual derivation from psychodynamic, behavioral, and developmental psychologies has been presented. We believe that our intervention contributed constructively to the baby's development and that of his next older brother. Significant problems do remain, however, and we will not be surprised if we hear from this family again.

References

Fraiberg, S., ed. (1980), *Clinical Studies in Infant Mental Health*. New York: Basic Books.

Greenspan, S., & Pollock, G. H., eds. (1980), *The Course of Life: Psychoanalytic Contributions Toward Understanding Personality Development*, Vol. 1. Washington, DC: U.S. Department of Health and Human Services.

Mahler, M., Pine, F., & Bergman, A. (1975), *The Psychological Birth of the Human Infant*. New York: Basic Books.

Part II:
Clinical Responses to Infants and Toddlers in Risky Environments

The development of an infant or toddler may be placed in jeopardy by the child's caregiving environment itself. Some parents are too overwhelmed by immediate demands or personal difficulties to respond adequately to an infant's needs. Some infants and toddlers have no permanent family, natural or adoptive, at all.

The chapters by Fred Volkmar and Albert Solnit and by Jean Adnopoz describe efforts to support the development of infants and toddlers in troubled families. For the family described by Volkmar and Solnit, "stitches in time" have not been taken: the fabric of Charlene's family is rapidly unraveling. Adnopoz, on the other hand, reports on a community effort to strengthen and support parents so that they can nurture more effectively and, as a result, prevent out-of-home placement of children.

These two chapters focus on young children and parents in their interactions with the legal system, child protective services, and the overall service delivery system in a community, rather than with institutions that traditionally offer "clinical" services to families. Nevertheless, the four elements of clinical responses are very much in evidence in the work reported here.

A Conceptual Framework

The two chapters that follow introduce specific, precisely defined concepts to guide professional decision making. They also offer a broader philosophical framework in which to consider the responsibilities that families and communities have toward very young children.

Volkmar and Solnit, for example, use the phrase "psychological parent" to denote a person in whose care a child can feel valued and wanted. One cannot assume that a biological parent (of either sex) or a blood relative functions as a child's psychological parent. Rather, one must learn whether a child relies on a given adult for nurturance and support and turns to that adult for assistance and security in preference to others. To serve the best interests of the child, Volkmar and Solnit argue, the psychological parent should prevail in a custody dispute.

Volkmar and Solnit also introduce the concept of "the least detrimental alternative available" to a child. They recognize the frustration that infant–family practitioners, legal professionals, and administrators feel when resources to promote "the best interests" of a vulnerable child are not at hand. Yet there is always a least detrimental alternative available; choosing this may at a minimum provide some stability to a child. The costs of uncertainty and repeated disruptions, even when assumed in a well-meaning search for better solutions, can be devastating to a rapidly developing infant or toddler.

Volkmar and Solnit declare their preference for minimum state intervention into the privacy of a family. A preference for minimum intervention, however, by no means rules out community or state efforts to offer support to parents. In fact, timely, appropriate support may reduce the need for coercive state intervention. As described by Jean Adnopoz, the Coordinating Council for Children in Crisis developed its approach using several basic assumptions: (1) that in order to serve young children, the needs of their parents must be understood and met; (2) that family stressors often are both intrafamilial and environmental; (3) that empowering families both creates independence and makes community services more effective; (4) that coordination of available community services promotes effectiveness; (5) that all cases should be voluntary; and (6) that involvement of multiple funding sources in a project gives concrete evidence of a commitment to shared goals and responsibilities.

Responsiveness to Individual Needs

Clinicians accustomed to working with individual infants and families may tend to think of the legal system and large service delivery systems as equitable and impersonal at best, rigid and inhumane at worst. The chapter by Volkmar and Solnit, however, reveals an attention to the particularities of a case that is also part of the legal tradition. The court asks its clinician-consultants very specific questions: What is the emotional and psychological status of the child and of her father? Has there been neglect? Who functions as the psychological parent? What support would be available to the father to enable him to function adequately as a father? Only against this background is the final question posed: What placement would be in the child's best interest?

Given the court's assignment, the clinicians raise questions of their own. They wonder whether the infant in question has special needs, requiring extraordinarily skillful child care. They try to gauge a troubled young man's capacity to learn to parent. They acknowledge the existence of prejudice against single fathers as primary caregivers. They recognize the passage of time as the enemy of the child who is in an unresolved or stressful situation.

In her account of the Coordinating Council for Children in Crisis, Jean Adnopoz describes efforts to "ground goals of intervention in the parents' reality" (p. 130). The parent is a key decision maker on his or her behalf and an active participant in all stages of case planning. When parents agree to a referral to a parent aide program, they meet with a program supervisor in their home and are invited to identify specific issues they wish to address. At quarterly case conferences plans are reassessed. The parent controls the duration of the parent aide's placement. While the agency initially assumed that two years would be the maximum length of a parent aide's involvement with a family, the agency is willing to assign aides for longer periods if required.

The Helping Relationship

These two chapters raise fascinating questions about the ground rules and boundaries of helping relationships between parents and practitioners.

As consultants to the court, Volkmar and Solnit must explain important ground rules to Charlene's father at the very beginning of their contact with him. The usual rules of confidentiality do not apply, and the clinicians' recommendations to the court will be based on what they believe will be the child's best interest. When it is decided that the court evaluation will be extended as Charlene's father undertakes a program of rehabilitation, the clinicians can act only as "monitors" of progress rather than as providers of services. Despite, or perhaps because of these constraints, the evaluation process seems to serve as a significant catalyst for self-change in the father, perhaps providing him with a previously lacking sense of structure.

The Coordinating Council model stresses the importance of the voluntary commitment of parents to work with the agency because "families . . . would believe that the help offered could be useful in dealing with the problems facing them" (p. 122). Program philosophy aside, families who are referred to the program as a final step before a child is removed from the home do not use services well and generally drop out.

These two reports illustrate the ways in which families can be helped both by formal, relatively infrequent contact and by intense involvement in daily life. The clinician–consultants in the case described by Volkmar and Solnit maintain a certain distance from the family being evaluated; in contrast, the parent aides who form the backbone of the Coordinating Council program become very involved with families, "parenting the parents" in their own home environments. They are listeners, organizers, and role models; sharing information from their own life experiences is also part of their job. The Coordinating Council model also includes a management team which includes the parent, the aide, the aide's supervisor, and the referring worker. The team not only reviews plans and allocates work but also provides support for both the families and the professionals working within it.

The role of the referring agency or individual is also addressed in both chapters. In the case of Charlene and her family, the court referral is limited in scope but ultimately therapeutic. In the Coordinating Council model, the referring worker not only smoothes the family's introduction into the program during a home visit, but also becomes a member of the case management team.

The System of Care

As Volkmar and Solnit note, a number of opportunities had been lost, before they became involved with Charlene, to support the biological parents of this vulnerable infant or to provide her with a permanent adoptive home early in her life. They point out the dangers of searching for theoretically better solutions that are in reality unavailable, while an infant is denied a potentially permanent home. The case also reminds us that fragmentation is far from the sole problem of service systems: neglect can occur in foster care; prejudices may bias the judgments of service providers. On the positive side, the existence of a variety of service models and, possibly, even the differences in state practices that result from the federal system continually offer new opportunities for rehabilitation to a family like Charlene's. One wonders if a more integrated but more monolithic human services system would have "written off" both parents and child.

As its name suggests, the Coordinating Council for Children in Crisis represents an effort to bring services together on behalf of children and families in order to reduce the separations experienced by children like Charlene. The Council seeks to foster greater collaboration between public and private sector agencies, and to improve both treatment planning and service delivery. Interestingly, the model is conceptualized as a way of enhancing the effectiveness of existing programs, not supplanting them. Also significant is the understanding that the goals of protecting children from harm and enhancing their development can only be accomplished when parents and children are served together. Perhaps the most important aspect of the Coordinating Council "system" is the emphasis on enabling client families to gain understanding of community resources and to claim the services they require to achieve independence.

3

Wishing for the "Wisdom" of Solomon: Custody Issues in a Case of Failure to Thrive

Fred R. Volkmar, M.D., Albert J. Solnit, M.D.

The issues posed by custody disputes are among the most challenging ones that face clinicians, social service agencies, lawyers, and judges. The conflicting agendas on the part of all the parties concerned make such disputes extremely complicated except in the most amicable of situations. The magnitude of the problem is suggested by the doubled divorce rate over the past two decades. Subsequent remarriages are even more likely to end in divorce (Cherlin, 1981). Approximately 10 million school-age children are currently living in one-parent families (Houts, 1979; Kohn, 1979). While some children weather the storm of parental disharmony, legal proceedings, and subsequent custody arrangements relatively well, it is clear that as a group, children of divorced parents are overrepresented in mental health and child guidance clinics

Acknowledgments. The authors gratefully acknowledge the collaboration of Dr. Sally Provence and Mrs. Barbara Nordhaus. Some aspects of the case have been changed to protect patient confidentiality. This work was supported in part by the William T. Grant Foundation and NIMH Grant MH00418. An earlier version of this case was presented at the Annual Meeting of the National Center for Clinical Infant Programs in December 1983.

(Tuckerman and Regan, 1966; Kalter, 1977; Kalter and Rembar, 1981) even many years after the divorce has occurred. Professional consultation to the courts becomes even more difficult when the child who is the object of the dispute already manifests some vulnerability. The case we present here illustrates the complex issues posed by such consultation and made us wish on more than one occasion for the wisdom of Solomon. As the title of the chapter alludes to what may be the first recorded child custody dispute, it is appropriate for us to begin with a review of that case and the judge's decision, as a way of illustrating several principles that helped to guide us in the case we present.

As outlined in I Kings, two unmarried women came before King Solomon; each claimed to be the mother of a child. One mother alleged that she really was the mother and her baby had been taken to replace the other woman's child, who had died. The other woman disputed this allegation. The king, whose wisdom was legendary, threatened to divide the baby in half and determined that the mother who was willing to give up the child rather than have him killed was in fact the psychological parent. King Solomon was careful to determine which mother was the psychological parent. Furthermore, he carefully returned the child to this mother in the expectation that she would best serve the child's interest.

Several principles used by Solomon in his decision continue to guide our work for the courts in the evaluation of custody disputes (Goldstein, Freud, and Solnit, 1979a, b). We share a preference for minimum state intervention into the privacy of the family and for a timely resolution of custody disputes, to the extent that this is humanly possible. We attempt to be guided at all times by the child's best interest; that is, in the complex web of competing needs and claims by the various parties to any custody dispute we believe that the child's needs should be paramount. In this connection it is important to determine who functions as the child's psychological parent(s), that is, the parent(s) in whose care the child can feel valued and wanted. This person(s) need not, necessarily, be one of the biological parents.

In the case to be described we have attempted to be guided by the best interest of the child, or what is more realistically correct, the least detrimental alternative available to the child. Although we were not able to use Solomon's simple device in resolving the dispute, our work included an attempt to determine who functioned primarily as the psychological parent for the child involved.

Case Presentation

PROCESS OF REFERRAL

As often happens in complex and protracted legal proceedings the "facts of the case" became apparent only over the course of an intensive and somewhat prolonged evaluation, which indirectly had the effect of an intervention. At various points in the evaluation process critical clinical decisions about the direction of the evaluation were made. In presenting this case material we have, therefore, chosen to present the information in the sequence in which it became available to us rather than in a more traditional fashion. This method of presentation will illustrate the development of the case and, at various points, will allow us briefly to review those decisions which, with the wisdom of hindsight, seem important to the ultimate resolution of this case. This method of presentation will, we hope, illustrate the complex and difficult task that clinicians face in providing expert opinions about custody issues.

The case of Charlene Daniels, age 13 months, first came to our attention when we received a request for an evaluation from the Connecticut Superior Court for Juvenile Matters to aid the court in a determination of two pending legal actions—coterminous petitions of neglect and for termination of parental rights. These actions were being vigorously contested by Charles Daniels, age 20. Although he had never married the child's mother, he was acknowledged to be Charlene's biological father. The biological mother, Laura Sutton, age 19, had requested that Charlene be placed for adoption and, at this stage of the proceedings, was not actively involved in the litigation over Charlene's placement. At the time that this court order was received Charlene resided in a foster home in Connecticut where she had been voluntarily placed by the father when she was 10 months of age.

Some limited historical information, furnished to the court by the state agency involved, was available to us at the time of the initial court order:

HISTORY OF THE CHILD

Charlene was born in a hospital in another state. She was a full-term healthy baby, the product of a presumably normal gestation and delivery, and weighed 5 pounds, 10 ounces at birth. She was readmitted to the same hospital three months later weighing 8 pounds, 10 ounces for evaluation of unexplained weight loss and dehydration. Although Charlene was rapidly rehydrated and discharged she was readmitted within a week with a diagnosis of pneumonia, was treated for this condition with antibiotics, did well in the hospital, and was again discharged to her biological mother. At 8 months of age she was hospitalized for gastroenteritis and inadequate weight gain. Her weight at the time of this admission was 11 pounds, and a diagnosis of failure to thrive was made. It was reported that during this hospitalization intensive efforts had been made to work with the mother and child, new formulas had been tried, and the staff were optimistic about the child's future growth and development. After a two-week hospitalization she was again discharged to her mother, but within a month the mother voluntarily placed Charlene for adoption with a private agency, saying that she was unable to care for the child adequately because of the persistent difficulties with feeding and poor weight gain. The mother also indicated that she was unaware of the location of the father, who, she said, had abandoned her and Charlene two months after the baby's birth. Within a week of being placed in foster care by the adoption agency, Charlene was again hospitalized for two weeks for gastroenteritis and further weight loss. On discharge from the hospital at age 9 months she was committed temporarily to the adoption agency's care and placed in an institution for children awaiting adoptive placement.

In the meantime the father learned of the placement and pending adoption and, to gain custody, went from Connecticut to the distant state where Charlene was living. Concurrently, the paternal grandmother requested, on her son's behalf, a voluntary foster placement in Connecticut, since she felt that he would be unable to care for the child immediately.

Even though the adoption agency vigorously contested Mr. Daniels's application for custody on the grounds of Charlene's fragile health and his history of abandonment, and recommended termination of his parental rights, the judge was persuaded to award custody to Mr. Daniels. Mr. Daniels's poignant statement in court of his desire to have Charlene returned to his care, and his assertion that he and his mother would care for the child seem to have influenced the judge's decision.

On the day of his return to Connecticut, Mr. Daniels left Charlene with her maternal grandmother. On the day of his arrival he officially requested a voluntary foster placement in this state. The state Department of Children and Youth Services (DCYS) drew up a detailed social service agreement, which Mr. Daniels signed and which stated clearly that the state agency would be guided by what it believed would be Charlene's best interest. Allegedly, other than mentioning her obviously small size, Mr. Daniels was unaware of Charlene's medical history from the time of his departure from Charlene and her mother. Furthermore he had made no attempt to elicit this information and it became available only when past medical records were requested. Charlene was placed in foster care within a week of her arrival in Connecticut. At the time of this placement, the maternal grandmother informed the agency that Mr. Daniels had a history of various legal difficulties and alcoholism and that she was not optimistic regarding his capacity to care for the child.

Despite his strong efforts to secure custody, once Charlene was placed in a foster home in Connecticut Mr. Daniels's visits to see her were, at best, sporadic. The foster home was thirty miles from his residence, and he was unable to drive since his driver's license had been revoked following a conviction for driving while intoxicated. The worker on the case encouraged Mr. Daniels to be more regular in his visitation, and several weeks after the initial placement Mr. Daniels did take Charlene for a weekend visit. However, the foster parents informed the state Department of Children and Youth Services that Charlene had subsequently been returned to them with multiple bruises, dried feces on her clothing, and car grease in her hair. The DCYS worker learned that Charlene had slept with her father on the floor during her visit to him and that she had helped him "work on some cars." This allegation of physical abuse/neglect was investigated, a process that was associated with Mr. Daniels's failure to visit Charlene for over a month. At the time of his next visit he was informed that he could visit Charlene only in the foster home and in the presence of the foster parents. At the

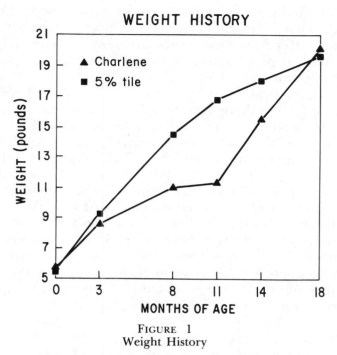

FIGURE 1
Weight History

same time the petitions of neglect and termination of parental rights were filed by DCYS. Mr. Daniels was informed of these proceedings and of his right to an attorney.

At no time since her original placement with the adoption agency at age 10 months did Charlene have any contact with her biological mother. Ms. Sutton had made no attempt to contact Mr. Daniels, his family, the state agency, or her own mother, who lived in Connecticut.

The court's request to our agency for this evaluation was quite detailed; it asked us to address the following questions: (1) Would Charlene's interests be best served by returning her to her father's care, by continuing the present arrangement (i.e., foster care) with supervised visitation, or by terminating parental rights? (2) If parental rights were terminated, what type of disposition would be in Charlene's best interest? (3) To what extent did the father suffer from a psychiatric disability, and how did this disability, if present, interfere with his capacity to parent and to profit from treatment?

In preparation of our study, we considered several questions. Was there already sufficient information available to make a determination of what course of action would be in the child's best interest? Would the father be able to take adequate care of her? He appeared to have had little contact with the child and none with the mother for several months after the child's birth. Furthermore, Charlene already exhibited evidence of vulnerability. We wondered whether she had special needs requiring extraordinarily skillful child care. The historical information available to us at this point made us skeptical about the father's interest in Charlene or his ability to parent even a normal infant. The court's detailed charge to us as consultants to the court highlighted these issues.

HISTORICAL INFORMATION REGARDING THE PARENTS
(Furnished by the courts and DCYS)

The salient points in the information provided us by the state child welfare agency as we began our contact were these: Mr. Daniels, age 20, was the second of two sons who had developed normally in the first years of life. Little was known of the extended family history. His parents had separated, as a result of his father's alcoholism, when Mr. Daniels was quite young. He had attended local public schools, where his academic performance had been poor; he had completed only the eighth grade. Mr. Daniels's adolescence was stormy. At age 15 he fathered twin boys, who were placed for adoption. His mother's attempts to encourage counseling were not successful, and he left her home at age 16 after an argument with her. At that time he was doing poorly in school, had a severe drinking problem, and had had several encounters with the juvenile justice system regarding charges of car theft, burglary, and assault and he had been placed on probation. After leaving home, Mr. Daniels met Laura Sutton, the woman who was to become Charlene's mother.

At this point, after an absence of many years, Mr. Daniels's father returned and indicated that he would be leaving to go to another state to find work. Mr. Daniels had not seen his father for some years but decided to accompany him. He was soon joined by Ms. Sutton. Although Mr. Daniels repeatedly attempted to secure employment he was not successful, in part because of his limited education and in part because of his continuing alcoholism.

Laura Sutton, Charlene's mother, was one year younger than Charles Daniels. She was a Connecticut native and the older of two children. She reportedly developed normally in the first years of life, but when she was 6 years of age, her father was killed in an industrial accident. His death seemed to have been a major blow to the development of Ms. Sutton, who had had a particularly strong relationship with her father. After his death she exhibited academic and behavioral problems at school and at home for the first time. She was frequently a truant and had many pitched battles with her mother. She became sexually active and began abusing herself with drugs and alcohol. She met and became intimate with Charles Daniels and followed him to another state when he left Connecticut to join his father.

At first things seemed to go well for the couple. Both Mr. Daniels and Ms. Sutton felt independent of their parents for the first time and were comfortable with their arrangement. They discussed marriage but never followed through. Ms. Sutton secured employment as a waitress and began to support both Mr. Daniels and herself, as his job opportunities proved limited. Within several months she was pregnant with Charlene. Neither she nor Mr. Daniels had used birth control. Though they were initially quite pleased with the pregnancy, Ms. Sutton experienced almost constant nausea, and felt increasingly frustrated, overwhelmed, and ill. During this time her relationship with Mr. Daniels deteriorated. He began to drink more heavily. Ms. Sutton worked throughout her pregnancy. When Charlene was born, both parents' names were listed on the birth certificate.

The period after Charlene's birth was a time of great stress for Ms. Sutton, who was supporting Mr. Daniels and the baby financially as well as taking care of the baby. Her anger and frustration increased over the two months following Charlene's birth; Mr. Daniels's drinking and unemployment persisted. The couple's relationship deteriorated, and, at Ms. Sutton's request, was terminated. Mr. Daniels returned to Connecticut, where he lived from time to time with family members, and where he was arrested for driving under the influence of alcohol.

After Mr. Daniels's departure, Ms. Sutton continued to work, placing Charlene in a number of different day care arrangements. Most of these were terminated because Charlene was noted to be overly fussy and demanding. Ms. Sutton received state assistance during this time to help pay for Charlene's day care, but when an investigation revealed that she had been working and had obtained this assistance fraudulently, she was threatened with legal charges and possibly imprisonment. She was forced to support herself and the baby from her own meager income and to repay the state for past support. This was a period of great stress and crisis, and Ms. Sutton appears to have had no timely assistance available to her.

Charlene's frequent illnesses and poor weight gain were extremely stressful for Ms. Sutton, who increasingly viewed Charlene as a hindrance and "like her father." The absence of a stable relationship with a man was also extremely frustrating for Ms. Sutton, until she met another man when Charlene was 6 months old, and moved in with him. While this man was able to provide some support for her and Charlene this relationship was also stormy. Ms. Sutton began extensive illicit drug use.

As indicated earlier, after Charlene's hospitalization at age 9 months the mother decided to place her for adoption and stated that she was unable to care for her child. She did not contemplate asking Mr. Daniels to assume custody, did not inform him of Charlene's placement, and remained angry and bitter about his perceived failings as a provider and father. Subsequent to the placement for adoption Ms. Sutton was not involved with Charlene. She did not visit her in any of the subsequent placements, and, when informed of the petition for termination of Mr. Daniels's parental rights, expressed interest only in whether she would have to appear in court.

In summary, the information provided us at the time of initial referral, before any examination of the involved parties, was that this 13-month-old girl with a history of failure to thrive requiring three hospitalizations; of multiple foster placements; and of multiple caregivers since birth, was the object of a dispute between the biological father and the State of Connecticut. The information provided us by the Department of Children and Youth Services suggested that the father was an immature, alcoholic young man with a history of multiple arrests, who had had little contact with the child from the time she was 2 months of age until she was 10 months old. Since he was awarded custody on her return to Connecticut at that time, he had had only sporadic contact with the child. There was also the suggestion that he had neglected or actually abused Charlene while she was in his care. The biological mother was in favor of an adoptive placement and had no continuing contact with the child. The court order asked us to evaluate the psychological and emotional status of both the child and her father. We were further asked to determine whether there had been neglect, who functioned as the psychological parent(s), what support would be available to the father to enable him to function adequately as a father, and what placement would be in the child's best interest.

In response to the court order, an extensive and usually prolonged evaluation was conducted over a period of several months. This evaluation consisted of repeated individual examinations of both Charlene and her father, including two separate developmental evaluations, individual interviews with the father, and joint interviews with the father and his mother. After the conclusion of this evaluation, a meeting with the biological mother was arranged at her request. As noted subsequently, the process of evaluation became an intervention in and of itself. This turn of events was, in part, the result both of the clinical evaluation and the protracted nature of the legal proceedings.

DEVELOPMENTAL EXAMINATION OF CHARLENE

At the time of the initial evaluation of Charlene she was 14 months of age. She was accompanied to the examination by her new foster parents, having been moved from her first Connecticut foster home after questions of neglect in that foster home were raised by both Mr. Daniels and the DCYS worker. Mr. Daniels had alleged that these foster parents, who had reported him for neglecting Charlene during a visit, were, in fact, themselves neglectful. While the worker was initially skeptical of Mr. Daniels's report, his impression was confirmed by the worker during an unscheduled visit to the foster home which resulted in Charlene's transfer.

The Yale Developmental Schedules were used to assess Charlene's development. She appeared to be small for her age and her weight was, in fact, less than the third percentile for her age. It was no surprise, given her history, that development was delayed and disturbed. Her gross motor skills were not yet at the one-year level, though fine motor skills were less delayed and closer to age level. Significant scatter was evident in her adaptive or problem-solving skills, and in her language. She was inhibited by new materials and had to be approached very carefully to avoid upsetting her. The level of social interaction was also delayed and characterized by inhibition, tension, and anxiety. Her foster mother described her as an anxious, easily disturbed child who preferred to spend much of her time alone and who engaged in self-stimulatory activities. The foster mother appeared to relate appropriately and sensitively to Charlene and seemed attuned to her needs. She was willing to tolerate Charlene's "fussiness" and her slow pace during feedings. She reported that Mr. Daniels visited occasionally and she seemed committed to helping him learn to care for Charlene. She noted, however, that he often depended on her for guidance and seemed rather anxious in his interactions with Charlene. His anxiety seemed to make visits with Charlene go badly, and she was generally irritable during and after his visits. Our consultation with Charlene's pediatrician revealed that she had continued to gain weight poorly, was often troubled with diarrhea, and continued to be a fussy eater. She responded to stressful events or disruptions in daily routine by refusing food. Thus, psychological reactions to stress were combined with developmental delays and psychological pain. The foster mother clearly stated that she would not be able to contemplate adopting Charlene.

EXAMINATION OF MR. DANIELS

At the beginning of our contact with Charles Daniels the ground rules were explained to him in some detail;

that his interviews with us were being done at the request of the court; that the usual rules of confidentiality did not apply; and that we would, in the end, make our recommendations based on what we believed would be Charlene's best interest. We also reviewed with him the information previously furnished to us. While he confirmed, in general, the history that had been provided to us by the court, he adamantly denied having ever abused or neglected Charlene. Rather, he insisted that his own lack of knowledge of young children's needs, his own conflict-ridden experience with his own father, and his very real problems with earning a living and alcoholism had made it difficult for him to assume a parental role.

Mr. Daniels told us that during the months since his return to Connecticut with Charlene he had continued to live a disorganized existence, relying on family and friends for support and assistance. He was also able to discuss his growing awareness of his own alcoholism. He had continued to drink heavily on occasion, particularly when overwhelmed by emerging feelings of frustration over his inability to care for Charlene or by anxiety about potential legal termination of his parental rights. Mr. Daniels denied other psychiatric problems and indeed had never participated in any attempts at counseling or psychotherapy.

Mr. Daniels described Charlene in a warm and appropriate way. While aware of her difficulties with poor weight gain and her developmental lags he seemed clearly committed to regaining custody. Over the month prior to our contact he had made some efforts to improve his life situation; he had secured employment and had arranged to live with family members nearer to Charlene.

During this initial interview Charles Daniels impressed us as an anxious and engaging young man who looked younger than his age. No thinking disorder was evident; he described himself and his life situation in appropriate ways. He did appear to be clinically depressed, relying on alcohol as a form of "self-medication." He had some insight into his difficulties, although he tended to blame the realities of his life history and current situation, as well as the adversarial nature of the court proceeding, for some part of his problems. Most important, Mr. Daniels appeared to be genuinely concerned for Charlene's welfare. He was obviously quite attached to her, although it was not clear to what extent this attachment could help motivate him to change. Initially, we estimated that he would not immediately be able to resume Charlene's care and that it was quite possible that he would never be able to do so. However, at this point a decision to conduct a more extensive evaluation, consisting in part of a trial of parental rehabilitation, was instituted. Several factors contributed to this decision.

It was clear that Mr. Daniels was attached to Charlene, that he was sufficiently motivated to engage in a program of rehabilitation, and that he had already made some efforts in this direction. It also appeared that Mr. Daniels would be a good candidate for professional counseling focused on his alcoholism and depression. Mr. Daniels's belief that he had been dealt with unfairly by the "system" appeared to have some basis in reality. He believed, with some justification, that the worker assigned to his case was biased against him because of her feeling that as an unmarried father he was not a suitable caretaker for Charlene. He said, "If I was an unmarried mother everyone would be trying to help me." At the same time we were cognizant of Charlene's needs. Unfortunately, the current foster parents, who related appropriately and warmly to Charlene, were not able to contemplate adoption, though they were willing to continue to care for her as foster parents. The litigation of the case had proven to be fairly lengthy and it was not clear when a decision regarding the child's eventual legal status would be forthcoming. Thus the "least detrimental alternative" appeared to be to maintain Charlene in the good care of the foster family, and to attempt to facilitate Mr. Daniels's rehabilitation.

INTERVENTION PROGRAM

We provided the court with an initial assessment of both Charlene and her father and our plan to help Mr. Daniels rehabilitate himself as a parent. In our letter to the court and in our discussion with Mr. Daniels we emphasized that we could act only as "monitors" of his progress and could not, in our role as consultants to the court, act to provide the various rehabilitation services directly. Mr. Daniels and the DCYS worker agreed with this plan. Over the next several months, Mr. Daniels engaged in an extensive, multifaceted, intervention program. He began an intensive alcohol treatment program and began to attend meetings of Alcoholics Anonymous on a regular basis; he maintained regular visitation with Charlene, and accompanied her to pediatric visits. During visits with Charlene he was helped to have a more realistic sense of her developmental needs, to work on basic parenting skills, and to assume increasing responsibility for her care. The foster mother was particularly helpful in this process. Mr. Daniels met with us many times over the course of the next several months, often alone but occasionally with Charlene and/or his own mother. During visits to us with his mother, Mr. Daniels and his mother explored various aspects of their relationship. Mrs. Daniels became more directly supportive of her son and granddaughter, eventually agreeing to provide both social and financial assistance.

Of interest to us was that the evaluation process served as a significant catalyst for self-change by Mr. Daniels. He clearly understood that our contact with him was being performed at the request of the court and in response to the court's order. The nature of the evaluation, the principles guiding our ultimate recommendations to the court (i.e., Charlene's best interest), and the unusual nature of our relationship with him (i.e., as consultants to the court) seemed to provide him with a sense of structure which had previously been lacking in his efforts to rehabilitate himself. He became increasingly responsible and capable, both as a person and as a parent. Though brief periods of regression were noted, on the whole he made significant progress over the course of the next three to four months. At our request he was allowed to take Charlene for increasingly long visits. He maintained sobriety, continued to work steadily, and developed an increasing sense of confidence in his capacity to parent. Gradually he developed a realistic plan for Charlene's care. After an extended visit with Charlene, it became apparent that she could be returned safely to her father's care on a trial basis.

Charlene was seen for another developmental examination at 17 months of age, when a return to her father's custody was deemed possible. At 17 months, though she remained a sensitive, easily upset child, she functioned appropriately in all aspects of her development. Gross and fine motor skills were at or above age level. Her language, problem-solving, and social skills had also improved and were at or close to levels expected for her age. Charlene was more obviously affectionate at this time. She was less likely to be a "fussy" eater, and her weight had surpassed the fifth percentile for her age. She had improved in all domains during the three months between her evaluations.

An out-of-court settlement was reached according to which Charlene was returned to her father's care on a trial basis. In the intervening months the biological mother, Ms. Sutton, returned to Connecticut and initially offered to testify against Mr. Daniels in court. When it became apparent that custody would be awarded him Ms. Sutton requested visitation rights. The court asked us to make a recommendation about the appropriateness of such visitation. After a meeting with Ms. Sutton and her mother it was clear that a desire to continue her stormy relationship with Mr. Daniels was a significant element in her wish for visitation. She made it quite clear that she would not contemplate requesting custody of Charlene. Our recommendation to the court was that it would be in the child's best interests to have the custodial parent determine visitation.

Since he was awarded custody when Charlene was 18 months old, Mr. Daniels has had one follow-up visit; he was accompanied by Charlene, who was then 23 months of age. Charlene related warmly to her father. It was clear that he functioned as her parent in all respects. She relied on him for nurturance and support, turned to him in preference to other adults for assistance, and continued to do well developmentally, though at times of stress she continued to be a fussy eater. Subsequent follow-up suggests that Charlene's growth and development are proceeding normally. She continues to have a strong primary relationship with her father.

Discussion

Several aspects of this case are noteworthy. The biological father, not the mother, was requesting custody. He suffered from a variety of psychological problems, legal difficulties, and alcoholism. The court's order for evaluation served as a catalyst for significant change. Finally, the child who was the object of the legal dispute had already exhibited some vulnerability in her failure to thrive, with recurrent gastrointestinal symptoms and eating problems.

Failure to thrive is a relatively common pediatric problem accounting for 1 to 5 percent of hospital admissions (Shaheen, Alexander, Truskowsky, and Barbero, 1968; Hanaway, 1976) and may be characterized as a decrement in progressive weight gain with subsequent changes in other aspects of physical growth (e.g., head circumference and length). A variety of other developmental and emotional changes in infants with failure to thrive are often noted as well. They have been reported to exhibit a variety of unusual behaviors; for example, "radar gaze," vigilance, diminished vocalizations, deviant patterns of social interaction, and/or unusual postures (Leonard, Phymes, and Solnit, 1966; Krieger and Sargent, 1966; Barbero and Shaheen, 1967; Rosen, Loeb, and Jura, 1980). Similarly, caretakers have been noted to exhibit a variety of psychiatric and psychosocial problems including depression, hostility, and impulsivity (Leonard et al., 1966; Evans, Reinhard, and Succop, 1972). Mothers of such infants may themselves have had disturbances in early childhood. In many cases, though certainly not all, significant psychosocial stressors are present.

Various diagnostic distinctions within this group of infants have been made (Goldbloom, 1982), though the most robust one has been that between organic failure to thrive (i.e., an organic "cause" for weight deceleration is identified) and nonorganic failure to thrive. Physical causes for failure to thrive include various endocrinological, gastrointestinal, central nervous system disorders, and chronic diseases, such as cystic fibrosis. However in as many as 55 percent of cases (Sills, 1978) no demonstrable organic cause for the growth disturbance can be identified. While cases of nonorganic failure to thrive have been most commonly attributed to various forms of maternal deprivation and deviance in maternal–infant bonding, an irritable, overly active, or difficult-to-soothe infant might also reasonably be expected to at times contribute to his or her own malnutrition (Kotelchuck and Newberger, 1983). Woolston (1983) has argued that nonorganic failure to thrive is a heterogeneous syndrome composed of at least three groups of children; those with reactive attachment disorders of infancy, those with simple calorie-protein malnutrition, and those with pathological food refusal. Practically, the differentiation of cases of organic versus nonorganic failure to thrive is problematic since many infants without demonstrable organic involvement will actually lose weight while hospitalized (Glaser, Heagerty, Bullard, and Pivchik, 1968) and the discovery of organic disease associated with the weight loss does not rule out a significant nonorganic component (Berwick, 1980). The relative contribution of maternal versus infant behavior in such cases has been the subject of much controversy. Some investigators have suggested that poor growth will result, even in the face of adequate nutrition, in the absence of proper emotional nurturance (Spitz, 1945) while others have suggested that caloric intake (regardless of emotional status) determines weight gain (Whitten, Petit, and Fischoff, 1969).

In Charlene's case, weight loss and subsequent failure to gain weight initially followed periods of apparent physical illness. Subsequently, however, the infant's difficulties with food refusal and feeding appeared to relate more directly to psychosocial factors arising from difficulties in the infant–adult relationship. Despite early attempts to promote better mother–child interaction the feeding difficulties intensified. Only when placed in an appropriately nurturing foster home did Charlene's weight gain begin to accelerate. Even at that time she remained vulnerable to disruption of eating patterns in response to environmental events.

The father's attempt to assume custody was also unusual. Typically in divorce actions, especially where infants are concerned, the father becomes the noncustodial parent. In this role he may respond in a variety of ways to the problems entailed in being a "part-time" parent (Wallerstein and Kelly, 1980; Hetherington, Cox, and Cox, 1982). Much less is known about the experience of fathers

as custodial parents (see Pruett [1980], Emery, Hetherington, and Dilalla [1984] for reviews). Mr. Daniels's history
of dependency and delinquency was less important per se
than his capacity to learn to parent.

In Charlene's first year, her experiences with the multiple caregivers and the transfer from one state to another
after the biological mother terminated her parental rights,
increasingly eroded Charlene's best interests. She became
a more vulnerable child. It was at times difficult for us to
focus on what opportunities remained for Charlene instead of on what she could or should have had earlier in
her experience. Alternatives became less and less promis-
ing and attractive, but there always remained, however, a
least detrimental alternative. As much as we could regret,
soft-heartedly, how unfair life had been to Charlene, it
was essential for her that we the child development experts
recommend, in a hard-headed way, the best of what alternatives were open to her (Goldstein et al., 1979a,b).

In this case we believed that the least detrimental alternative from the child's point of view was to attempt to
engage the biological father in a program of rehabilitation.
Obviously, had we been consulted at the time of Charlene's
original placement in foster care by her mother, we might
well have recommended termination of parental rights,
given the father's lack of a relationship with the child and
his past history. However, the realities of Charlene's situation and our study of her impaired father suggested that
a trial of parental rehabilitation offered the best possibility
of promoting the child's future growth and development.
In and of itself, the "blood tie" made no difference in our
evaluation–intervention program. What was important
was the willingness and ultimately the proven capacity of
the father to act as Charlene's caregiver, and to demonstrate that *he* wanted her more than anyone else who was
immediately available.

Certainly the initial historical information given to us made us skeptical of his capacity to parent this vulnerable infant. One might well ask why, in this case, the father was able to profit from our intervention. A combination of factors appears to have been important in enabling Mr. Daniels to assume his role as Charlene's parent. The process of the evaluation had an organizing influence on Mr. Daniels. His awareness of the urgency of the situation, of our work as consultants to the court, and his awareness of his own difficulties helped Mr. Daniels fruitfully engage with us in our attempt to unite him with his daughter. Additionally, Mr. Daniels mobilized a variety of other services and social supports in the course of the evaluation. These included alcohol treatment and vocational rehabilitation programs, the foster mother, the pediatrician, and his own family as sources of information and support. Mr. Daniels's own feeling that the evaluation process was enabling him to function in a more organized and effective manner was also important.

Because of failures in our efforts to provide children with the continuity of sustained affectionate relationships without the corrosive passage of time, clinical and legal experts are often confronted with difficult assessments and choices. In Charlene's case it was too late to provide her biological mother with the supportive services that might have enabled her to care for her daughter in a manner that prevented failure to thrive and that would have precluded giving her up for adoption. It was too late to give Charlene a better alternative than coming to Connecticut (i.e., adoption in the state of her birth, which would have prevented multiple moves and placements). It was not legally feasible to carry out an immediate adoptive placement once Charlene was brought to Connecticut.

Instead, when the court asked for our consultation, we found an unstable, impaired biological father who had legal custody and wanted Charlene; an initial foster placement in Connecticut that was damaging to the child; and a second placement with foster parents who did not wish to adopt Charlene but who helped the child and her biological father to come together on a sound permanent basis.

Earlier, there had been at least two, and probably three alternatives potentially better than the one we recommended and monitored, but they were no longer available. Further erosion of Charlene's potential would probably have occurred if efforts had been made to resurrect these alternatives; in other words, if implementation of the least detrimental alternative was deferred while a search for a theoretically better, but unavailable practical solution was undertaken. The delays associated with such a process would have compounded Charlene's tragedy.

While we may have wished for the wisdom of Solomon as we worked with Charlene and her parents, we realized that applying psychoanalytic and developmental knowledge to child placement conflicts would never yield an instant "test," like Solomon's through which Mr. Daniels could prove his love, fidelity, and competence as a father. We needed to avoid "studying what is measurable but not meaningful" (Charney, 1983). We tried, rather, to keep in mind our desire for minimal intrusion into the privacy of the family and our paramount concern for the best interests of the child. We looked for a way to apply the principle that a child should be placed permanently as soon as is feasible with adults who want the child and who can provide the *sustained* affectionate care that each child needs. Consultation to parents and courts in custody disputes requires considerable expertise and skill; a commitment to the value of continuity of care; and an ability to integrate scientific and clinical information. All of our efforts are directed toward facilitating, to the greatest extent possible, the future development of each child.

References

Barbero, G., & Shaheen, E. (1967), Environmental failure to thrive: A clinical view. *J. Pediatr.*, 71:639–644.

Bell, L. S., & Woolston, J. L. (1985), The relationship of weight gain and caloric intake in infants with organic and nonorganic failure to thrive syndrome. *J. Amer. Acad. Child Psychiat.*, 24:447–452.

Berwick, D. (1980), Nonorganic failure to thrive. *Pediatr. in Rev.*, 1:265–270.

Charney, E. (1983), Secondary care: The role of the community hospital in pediatrics. *Amer. J. Dis. Child.*, 137:902–906.

Cherlin, A. L. (1981), *Marriage, Divorce, Remarriage.* Cambridge, MA: Harvard University Press.

Emery, R. F., Hetherington, E. M., & DiLalla, L. F. (1984), Divorce, children, and social policy. In: *Child Development Research and Social Policy*, ed. H. W. Stevenson & A. E. Siegel. Chicago: University of Chicago Press.

Evans, R., Reinhard, J., & Succop, R. (1972), Failure to thrive: A study of 45 children and their families. *J. Amer. Acad. Child Psychiat.*, 11:440–457.

Fischoff, J., Whitten, D., & Pettit, M. (1971), A psychiatric study of mothers of infants with growth failure secondary to maternal deprivation. *J. Pediatr.*, 79:209–215.

Glaser, H., Heagarty, M., Bullard, D., & Pivchik, E. (1968), Physical and psychological development of children with early failure to thrive. *J. Pediatr.*, 73:690–698.

Goldbloom, R. (1982), Failure to thrive. *Pediatr. Clin. N. Amer.*, 29:151–166.

Goldstein, J., Freud, A., & Solnit, A. (1979a), *Beyond the Best Interests of the Child.* New York: Free Press.

———— ———— (1979b), *Before the Best Interests of the Child.* New York: Free Press.

Hanaway, P. (1976), Failure to thrive: A study of 100 infants and children. *Clin. Pediatr.*, 9:96–99.

Hetherington, E. M., Cox, M., & Cox, R. (1982), Effects of divorce on parents and children. In: *Nontraditional Families*, ed. M. Lamb. Hillsdale, NJ: Lawrence Erlbaum.

Houts, P. L. (1979), The American family minus one. *Nat. Element. Princ.*, 59:10–11.

Kalter, N. (1977), Children of divorce in outpatient psychiatric population. *Amer. J. Orthopsychiat.*, 47:40–51.

———— Rembar, J. (1981), The significance of the child's age at the time of parental divorce. *Amer. J. Orthopsychiat.*, 51:85–100.

Kohn, S. (1979), Coping with family change. *Nat. Element. Princ.*, 59:40–50.

Kotelchuck, J., & Newberger, E. (1983), Failure to thrive: A controlled study of familial characteristics. *J. Amer. Acad. Child Psychiat.*, 4:322–328.

Krieger, I., & Sargent, D. (1967), A postural sign in the sensory deprivation syndrome in infants. *J. Pediatr.*, 70:332–339.

Leonard, M., Phymes, J., & Solnit, A. (1966), Failure to thrive in infants. *Amer. J. Dis. Child.*, 111:600–612.

Pruett, K. (1980), Infants of primary nurturing fathers. *The Psychoanalytic Study of the Child*, 38:257–277. New Haven, CT: Yale University Press.

Rosen, D., Loeb, L., & Jura, M. (1980), Differentiation of organic from nonorganic failure to thrive syndrome in infancy. *Pediatr.*, 66:698–704.

Shaheen, E., Alexander, D., Truskowsky, M., & Barbero, G. J. (1968), Failure to thrive: A retrospective study. *Clin. Pediatr.*, 7:255–260.

Sills, R. H. (1978), Failure to thrive: The role of clinical and laboratory evaluation. *Amer. J. Dis. Child.*, 132:967–969.

Spitz, R. A. (1945), Hospitalism: An inquiry into the genesis of psychiatric conditions in early childhood. *The Psychoanalytic Study of the Child*, 1:53–74. New York: International Universities Press.

Togut, M. R., Allen, J. E., & Lelchuchk, L. (1969), A psychological exploration of the non-organic failure to thrive syndrome. *Devel. Med. Child Neurol.*, 11:601–607.

Tuckerman, J., & Regan, R. A. (1966), Intactness of the home and behavioral problems in children. *J. Child Psychol. Psychiat.*, 7:225–233.

Wallerstein, J. S., & Kelly, J. B. (1980), *Surviving the Breakup: How Children Actually Cope with Divorce*. New York: Basic Books.

Whitten, C. F., Petit, M. G., & Fischoff, J. (1969), Evidence that growth failure from maternal deprivation is secondary to undereating. *J. Amer. Med. Assn.*, 209:1675–1682.

Woolston, J. L. (1983), Eating disorders in infancy and early childhood. *J. Amer. Acad. Child Psychiat.*, 22:114–121.

4

Reaching Out: The Experiences of a Family Support Agency

Jean Adnopoz, M.P.H.

Introduction

A decade after Helfer and Kempe (1968) identified the battered child syndrome and set into motion an eventual torrent of activity involving legislative mandates, child welfare practices, and the media, a Connecticut community utilized a grass-roots approach to build a voluntary program of support for families at risk. Initially spearheaded by a group of hospital volunteers, an effort to achieve a public and private sector coalition resulted in the creation of a new nonprofit community agency committed to strengthening and supporting troubled families and reducing the need for out-of-home placement of children.

In 1977, the Coordinating Council for Children in Crisis was incorporated in New Haven, Connecticut, for the primary purpose of developing and providing services to maintain children within their own homes with their primary caretaker (most frequently a biologic parent) and to avoid multiple separations from the parent and the problems arising from discontinuities of caregiving. Secondarily, the new agency sought to enhance collaboration between public and private sector agencies on behalf of abused, neglected, and at-risk children and their families for the purpose of improving coordination, treatment planning, and service delivery. Utilizing the experience of the Comprehensive Emergency Service Program (National Center for Comprehensive Emergency Services to Children, 1976) and the Lower East Side Family Union project (1976), the Coordinating Council developed a range of paraprofessional services for voluntary use by families whose own resources were insufficient for them to offer their children a consistently nurturing and safe environment. The maintenance of children in their own families or in long-term foster families was the agency's stated mission, and the agency expected to implement and use a range of interventions to reach its goal. The agency was prepared to be flexible and to respond on an individual basis to cases which were referred to it. It was willing to test models and make changes as its knowledge base expanded.

The agency chose as its service area a region consisting of the central city, New Haven, and nineteen nearby towns with both urban and suburban characteristics. The population to be served was poor, almost exclusively receiving welfare support from the Aid to Dependent Children program (AFDC), racially mixed, jobless, and with minimum education. The task of identifying and creating services which would allow the agency to attain its mission required that the Board and its Director think through a set of assumptions which would inform program development, offer coherence to the agency as a whole, and serve as guiding principles for present and future program expansion.

Faculty members of the Yale Child Study Center, community health and mental health professionals, and members of the Department of Children and Youth Services (DCYS) played critical roles as board members in formulating these principles and conceptualizing the programs which resulted:

The basic assumptions were these:

1. Understanding and meeting the needs of the parents of young dependent children would be an essential element of serving the children. Goals for service to children were both to protect them from harm and, beyond that, to positively enhance their development. Parents whose own basic needs had not been met would require support and assistance before they could be expected to successfully meet the needs of their children.

2. Family stressors often were both intrafamilial and environmental. To reduce family dysfunction effectively, major consideration had to be given to impacting on individual needs in areas such as housing, entitlements, nutrition, and education, as well as on a systems level. It was expected that the provision of concrete services to address these needs would enhance the utilization and effectiveness of the mental health services already available in the community.

3. It was felt that empowering client families to claim the benefits of community resources could make a difference not only in the utilization of services but in their effectiveness. The program hoped to create independence, not dependency, by providing an opportunity for clients to gain understanding of the various systems with which they interact and to feel more powerful in their transactions.

4. It was felt that coordination of available community services to individuals and families would promote their effectiveness. In this regard, the new agency should seek to implement only those additional programs which were not available elsewhere in the community and which did not fit the program mix of other agencies or institutions. The new agency should be sensitive to the territoriality of other programs in the community and seek to bring

these programs into the network rather than to compete with them. With scarce financial and human resources and ever increasing pressure on the system to provide service to the client population, it was in the interest of each agency in the community to be a collaborator and to define clearly its own area of interest and expertise.

5. Location of the program in the private sector could be an advantage because it would reduce the possibility of the perception of the agency as a coercive intervenor, as public programs often are considered, and would minimize the stigmatization of its clients. To foster client acceptance and commitment to working with the agency, all cases were to be voluntary; families themselves would believe that the help offered could be useful in dealing with the problems facing them.

6. The involvement of multiple funding sources in the program would have advantages beyond the important first step of realistic support: it would be evidence of a commitment on the part of each funding entity to the goals of coordination of service, as well as the acknowledgment of shared responsibility for children and families. The reduction of fragmentation was dependent upon such collaboration.

The Department of Children and Youth Services (DCYS) provided the funding for the first staff member, a coordinator, whose task was to create the agency's program in response to community needs but without the promise of any additional financial support. The staff member, who became the Agency's Executive Director, worked with a board which was representative of many of the existing children's programs to identity needed services, to seek funding sources, and to implement programs. The support and involvement of DCYS on both the state and regional level was critical to the success of the agency because it sanctioned worker involvement, gave validation to the program's goals and objectives, and smoothed the way for public–private collaboration on the local level.

Within one year of incorporation, the Coordinating Council was able to offer the following programs:

Interdisciplinary Case Consultation Teams
Parent Aides
Family Advocates
Community Education

Seven years later the range of service had expanded to include

Teaching Homemakers
Student Aides
Child Sexual Abuse Program
Project Home Share
Case Management Services
A Family Intervention Team

Initial funding from the State Department of Human Resources, Comprehensive Employment and Training Administration (CETA), a federal program which provided salary support for unemployed low-income persons willing to learn new skills with the expectation that they would then be qualified for permanent employment, and the Juvenile Justice commission, made possible the first of the agency's services. The Departments of Health and Mental Health, private foundations, and community contributions were added over the years to the list of funding resources which enabled the agency to continue to respond to the unmet needs of the community.

All programs described were offered to residents of the agency's South Central Connecticut region at no charge. Self-referrals were not accepted; in most programs clients were referred by other service providers, who were expected to have the potential client's permission to do so. This process helped to screen inappropriate clients and enlisted the referrer as part of the intervention team. Primary referral sources were the Department of Children and Youth Services, the welfare agencies, hospitals, mental health facilities, university clinics, and other social service agencies. More than 300 families received service during 1983 and 1984.

The agency was headed by an executive director, who reported to the board of directors and had overall responsibility for all programs, fiscal operations, including identification of funding sources, and future development. She was also the facilitator of the multidisciplinary teams.

Program coordinators reported to the executive director and had supervisory responsibilities for program sectors: In-Home Services, Case Management and Advocacy, Project Home Share, and Sexual Abuse Advocacy and Information.

In-Home Services

In-home services were provided by parent aides, teaching homemakers, student aides, and the family support service. The unit consisted of two supervisors, one of whom acted as coordinator, six full-time workers, graduate and undergraduate students from local colleges and universities, and volunteers who made a minimum commitment of ten hours per week.

The goal of the parent aide program was consonant with the agency's mission: to support and strengthen families so that they could nurture more effectively and, as a result, to prevent out-of-home placement. The in-home services were directed toward reducing intrafamilial stressors by long-term work with the parents, helping to meet parental needs, providing support and reinforcement for families, and coordinating the resources involved with the family.

Although this chapter focuses in detail upon the work of parent aides and teaching homemakers, student aides were valued components of in-home services. Student aides were university volunteers who functioned as friendly visitors for the children in families served by the in-home programs. This was the only Coordinating Council program designed to serve children directly. The students met their "littles" (the names used for the children with whom they worked) weekly during the academic year, taking them to special events and recreational activities, or spending a quiet time of conversation and tutoring. The student aides were treated as part of the agency team working with an individual family and benefiting from group supervision and training. Many of the approximately twenty students volunteering in the program continued their involvement throughout their university years. The agency provided funds to cover costs of activities and for a special excursion, usually to the Bronx Zoo, at the end of the academic year.

Parent Aides

In a typical year during the first decade of the Coordinating Council, seventy-nine families were served by the parent aide program of the Coordinating Council. In 44 percent of these families, neglect was the principal reason for referral; 37 percent of the families were considered to be at risk; 10 percent were referred for emotional abuse; and in 9 percent of the families, children were physically abused.

The placement of a parent aide was an opportunity to parent the parent, to offer the mother the assistance of an aide who represented the strengths of a good parent, trusting, accepting, nonjudgmental, and consistent. Aides were trained to act as role models for the parent, to offer support and encouragement. Parent aides worked with mothers in their own home environments, visiting at least once weekly for a period of two to three hours. The parent, the aide, the aide's supervisor, the referring worker, and other case-specific persons formed a management team which set the goals for the parent aide placement. In addition, this team reviewed and updated the quarterly case plan. The parent was a key decision maker on her or his own behalf and an active participant in all stages of case planning and problem identification. The parent also controlled the duration of the placement. Empowering the family to make responsible decisions on its own behalf was an important part of the work. Families who were reluctant to become involved or were referred to the program as a final step before a child was removed did not utilize the intervention well and generally dropped out.

The management team, itself, functioned as a "community of concern" (Young-Saxon, 1983), providing support for both the family and the professionals working within it. The management team called attention to the tasks that the family had chosen to accomplish and allocated the work in such a way as to minimize the tendency of parent aides to feel overburdened or solely responsible for the safety of the children. In fact, many members of the case specific teams reported feeling supported by it.

Parent aides became involved in the life of the family, acting as facilitators and organizers; going shopping, helping to take children to health and mental health appointments, accompanying parents to therapy, assisting families to work with other community agencies, identifying appropriate resources for child care and enrichment, and helping to create meaningful networks for the family. The aide was a good listener, available to parents, who often had no other person in whom they could trust and to whom they could confide the details of their lives. Families served by the parent aide program were largely poor; 85 percent were AFDC recipients, 6 percent were employed, and 9 percent received supplemental entitlements. Families were white, 48 percent; black, 42 percent; and Hispanic, 10 percent. These families had an average of 2.6 children per family. The age of the mothers ranged from 17 to 42 years; 38 percent were between 19 and 25 years, while 35 percent were between 25 and 30 years. There was a predominance of single parent families (89%). Only 11 percent of the families included two parents.

In more than 75 percent of the families referred to the Parent Aide program, one or more of the following were true:

1. The parent was overwhelmed by the circumstances of his or her life.
2. The parent had few, if any, positive interpersonal relationships.
3. The parent had experienced multiple rejections over time.
4. The parent had little or no understanding of the child's needs as separate from her or his own.
5. The parent was unable to manage the family without assistance.
6. The parent lacked an effective support system.
7. The parent had not had a positive relationship with other human service providers.

Providing adequate support to maintain the family as a unit required considerable energy and involvement; the agency initially assumed that two years would be the maximum length of parent aide cases. However, the assumption failed to recognize that there were some families who would require indefinite support, although the intensity of the intervention might lessen and the amount of time spent with the aide could be reduced. The fact that the agency was willing to assign parent aides to families for long periods of time when the case required it, demanded that attention be paid to those factors which made it possible for an aide to remain useful to the family.

Of primary importance was the type of person chosen to work as a parent aide. The fourteen parent aides originally hired by the Coordinating Council were CETA employees. They were exclusively women with no education beyond high school and little job experience. Many had spent their lives raising children, often under circumstances similar to those of our clients.

The agency sought candidates for the position who were warm, caring, and nonjudgmental. These women needed to be able to share information from their own life experiences and to have some positive memories of their child-rearing years. The agency offered these women regular supervision, an opportunity to develop marketable skills and increase their knowledge through weekly didactic training sessions, and provided a time each week for peer support and sharing.

Parent aides reported that a support group comprised of agency personnel (including the supervisor and the aide's peers, as well as case-specific professionals from the community) which mirrored the team supporting the family itself, was the most effective means of keeping the aide successfully involved in the long-term case. Continued training and opportunities to grow professionally added to the self-esteem of the parent aide and increased personal gratification in what was a particularly isolated and stressful work experience. Kempe warned that difficulties can arise when the aide receives too much gratification from overly dependent clients (Helfer and Kempe, 1968). The aide was assisted to separate her own needs from those of the client, to recognize client growth, to maintain realistic expectations, and to be satisfied with small changes. Although the goal of the intervention was to strengthen the family so that it could meet the needs of its own members, the parent aide could not go beyond the limits of current knowledge or the natural endowments of each family.

Families with young children were thought to be more likely to experience positive outcomes from their work with parent aides than families whose patterns of dysfunction had persisted for long periods. The program found that the mothers most likely to utilize the service effectively were those who were unsupported and overwhelmed during the child's infancy and early childhood and recognized that they could not manage successfully without assistance.

Professionals who referred cases for parent aide involvement were assumed to have explained the program carefully to the parent and to have elicited the parent's voluntary agreement to accept the intervention. Once a referral was made, a home visit was scheduled with the referrer and the parent aide supervisor. The referring person smoothed the transition to the new program and demonstrated that the program was, in fact, a collaboration in support of the family.

The supervisor used a structured interview format to enable the parents to identify specific problem areas. The parent was asked to specify which of the following presented difficulties: child care routine, specific child care functions, parent–child relationships, child management, housekeeping, budgeting and shopping, nutritional planning, personal hygiene, social isolation, family violence, substance abuse, medical care, mental health problems, educational problems, transportation, housing and utilities, and/or utilization of community resources. The information was used to develop and establish baseline data, against which the effectiveness of the intervention could be measured. The identified problem areas were reviewed at the case-specific conferences which were held quarterly, allowing for feedback which led to reassessment of the case plan. To maximize the parents' opportunity to experience success whenever possible, the goals of the intervention were grounded in the parents' reality and did not presume major changes in the functioning in the near term.

Without further research, we do not know if certain characteristics of the family are predictive of outcome. Approximately 20 percent of the cases accepted by the program and placed on the waiting list after the initial interview decided not to accept a parent aide when it was time to make the actual assignment. We do not know if these families found other services more easily accessible, if a need for immediate gratification made waiting impossible, or if family circumstances had been altered. There are many questions yet to be answered if resources are to be used most efficiently.

Case Studies

The following are case studies from the agency's records which illustrate the roles played by parent aides in families with infants and young children. The primary factors in determining the need for a parent aide have been the capacity of the parent to care for the child, the level of functioning of the parent, and the mother's desire to maintain the child in the home. The mothers described in this sample suffered chronic mental illness or possessed limited intelligence. These criteria for selection were necessary because the demand for service exceeded the resources available and served to eliminate less severe cases. Many of the children in these families would have faced out-of-home placement or possible parental neglect if a parent aide was not available. None of the parents requested placement for their children, nor was there any cause for the state to seek to intervene coercively at the time of the referral. Although none of these cases has been followed beyond termination, many children and parents showed marked improvement in functioning and appropriate utilization of their community resources at the time the case closed. However, not all families are able to nurture effectively even when the community provides a massive infusion of support. Such a case is also described.

CASE 1

Mr. and Mrs. A. A parent aide was placed with Mr. and Mrs. A at the request of the Visiting Nurse Association. The family consisted of three children aged 4 years, 3 years, and 9 months. Mrs. A, aged 34, had a history of depression, was significantly underweight, and slept excessively. The oldest child was subject to dizzy spells which were undiagnosed at the time of referral. Mother was in need of someone to help her manage her household and teach her basic child-rearing skills. Immediately prior to the placement of the aide, Mrs. A was treated at a psychiatric hospital, which endorsed the placement of the parent aide and also recommended that Mrs. A continue individual psychotherapy as an outpatient with her previous therapist. A visiting nurse was to continue helping mother with the care of her children on a weekly or bimonthly schedule. At the time that Mrs. A was discharged from the hospital and prepared to return home, her depression had lifted, she had gained 10 pounds, and was able to say that she liked herself for the first time in her life. The parent aide began work with mother immediately upon her hospital discharge. The areas identified by Mrs. A as most problematic were organizing her household, enrolling her children in appropriate day care programs, providing medical care for her children, establishing a weight gain program for herself, and shopping at the same time she had to care for her children.

The parent aide assigned to Mrs. A was a mature, empathetic, and caring woman who had four years of experience as a parent aide. She met Mrs. A's request for someone her own age or a little older. Her initial contacts with the family were home visits, during which she met Mr. A and other extended family members and became well acquainted with Mrs. A and her children. Seated at the kitchen table, they would discuss mother's feelings about the hospital stay, her relationship with her family, and her problems in taking care of her small children. According to the parent aide, at times Mrs. A appeared tense and anxious; at other times the whole family relaxed, laughing and playing together. Gradually mother revealed to the aide her sense of her inadequacy, her abusive relationship with her own mother, her guilt about doing things which satisfied only her own needs, such as getting away from her children for an hour or two, and concerns about her children's health.

The aide was instrumental in arranging a complete medical workup for the oldest child, who also received speech therapy prior to entering school. She helped mother enroll the baby in the same speech therapy program at the time of his second birthday, when he began to show signs of speech delay. She encouraged mother's active involvement in play with her children, took her to stores to shop for clothing and other items for them, and helped her to meet her own medical needs. The aide initiated toilet training for the baby at 28 months with mother's involvement.

After ten months of the parent aide placement, the visiting nurse was withdrawn from the case. The parent aide and the therapist became a support team for the mother. They met together periodically with mother and the parent aide supervisor, reviewing the treatment plan and assessing its effectiveness.

The parent aide had helped Mrs. A to become more actively involved in play with her children, to take pride in their appearance, to treat them affectionately, and also to set limits and encourage responsible behavior, such as putting toys away and being neat. The children had made good adjustments to school and had responded positively to the affection of mother and the parent aide.

Weekly visits to the home continued for 18 months, during which time substantive gains were made in improving Mrs. A's self-image. As she was encouraged to assert herself by taking control of her household and setting limits for her children, she was gradually able to make time for herself, take pride in herself and her surroundings, and function more independently. Mrs. A started a Bible study group in her own home and went to a church group regularly.

When termination of the parent aide began to be discussed, Mrs. A's initial reaction was, "I am going to get bad, so you won't have to go." Subsequent weekly meetings focused on mother's anxiety about managing on her own and how much the parent aide would be missed by all the family. Although termination has taken place, Mrs. A can request further contact if the pressures of managing her family become overwhelming once again.

CASE 2

Mr. and Mrs. W. Mr. and Mrs. W, aged 25, each intellectually limited, were the parents of two boys aged 28 months and 10 months when the case was referred by a Visiting Nurse Association (VNA) for a parent aide. When the aide was placed eight months later, the goals for the placement were assistance in child management, enrolling the children in a nursery school program, teaching some basic child development information, nutritional planning, and assistance in budgeting and shopping.

Both children were developmentally delayed; because the baby did not sit unaided at 10 months, the pediatrician had recommended additional stimulation. This was being provided by a staff member of an early stimulation program and was to end shortly. The VNA visited the family biweekly.

Mr. W was employed, and Mrs. W was responsible for the majority of the child care. She was socially isolated, with no friends, and had a limited knowledge of community facilities. Mrs. W did not drive, a fact that increased her isolation in the rural town in which they lived.

As the parent aide became involved in the life of the family, she began to take the family to visit the local library, especially the children's room, and the playground. These became important places where the children could work puzzles, be read to, or become familiar with equipment which until then had been unfamiliar and threatening. The aide encouraged Mr. W to give his wife driving lessons and took her to visit the Motor Vehicle Department.

The aide arranged a scholarship for the older child in a nursery school, but when the family decided to move to a neighboring town this could not be used. The ease with which the first school placement was achieved contrasted markedly with the difficulty that the aide faced in locating an appropriate day care placement in the family's new location. This time the pediatrician and the aide worked closely together to request a meeting of the Pupil Planning Team after a developmental evaluation by the pediatrician reaffirmed that the child would benefit from a structured group experience on a regular basis.

The school system responded positively to the results of pediatric evaluation and the gentle proddings of the parent aide to obtain an appropriate day care placement. The parents were interviewed and the child tested at home, and the recommendations resulted in the child's enrollment in an appropriate day care program at the expense of the town. The child made a very successful entry into school, much to the delight of his parents and the parent aide. With this step accomplished, the aide focused some of her attention on the older child's hearing problems, which had become noticeable and in which the pediatrician was taking an active interest. There was a possibility that the child's speech difficulties could be related to his hearing problems. Mrs. W was helped to maintain medication schedules for her children and to keep their medical appointments. When surgery was recommended to correct the hearing difficulties, the aide helped Mrs. W understand the procedure and what the benefits would be. In fact, the outcome was positive, and the child's speech and understanding improved rapidly. The pediatrician also recommended that the younger child be evaluated developmentally and that his hearing be tested as well.

The parent aide remained with this family for 15 months. During that time the children became familiar with a range of stimulating experiences, including numerous trips to the beach and to town which expanded their environment and increased their socialization skills.

Although mother was limited and unable to deal with abstract concepts, she was able to love her children and meet their basic needs; most importantly, she was able to make good use of the many supports that became available to her. The support of the pediatrician, the visiting nurse, and the "child find" resource who preceded the parent aide were essential in getting this family off to a positive start. However, this family will require ongoing support and assistance if the children are to reach their own maximum potential. Although the aide has terminated, it is hoped that the pediatrician and the school system will continue their collaboration so that the family's many gains can be sustained.

CASE 3

Janice G. Janice G was a 32-year-old, single woman who was hospitalized on a psychiatric ward two weeks prior to delivery of her only child. The referral to the parent aide program was made by a protective services worker one week after the child's birth. Ms. G was diagnosed as psychotic and was treated at the hospital for approximately one month while being started on medication. Her daughter was placed in foster care initially, but later returned to her parent's home with the help of a parent aide.

The first meeting between the aide and Ms. G took place in the hospital. At that time Ms. G expressed concern about plans for her to live with her own parents and revealed some anxiety about their reaction to the intrusion of herself and her baby into their home. It was agreed that the aide would help Ms. G with child care and nutrition and provide ongoing support in this stressful situation.

Prior to discharge from the hospital, Ms. G returned home several times on a pass and was able to establish contact with her baby. She looked forward to assuming responsibility for the child, although she expressed concern about the limitations the baby would impose on her freedom. Ms. G was a talented illustrator who took pride in her work and wanted to find a position as soon as possible.

Ms. G and her baby were reunited when the baby was 7 weeks old. The foster mother helped Ms. G to understand the baby's routine and became another important resource for the family.

Accepting the reality of her situation was difficult for mother; she wished that the baby's father, who became a regular visitor to the home, would resume his relationship with her. The parent aide was able to serve as a confidante, a thoughtful listener. The aide encouraged Ms. G to remain in therapy, supported her desire to find housing separate from her elderly parents, and helped her through a dispute between the welfare office and the putative father involving support payments.

When the baby was 6 months old, the child protective worker closed the case, having found the baby to be well cared for and with appropriate development. More terminations were likely in the near future; the parent aide would be leaving the program, and the only support person continuing with Ms. G would be her therapist. The parent aide program facilitated a case conference with Ms. G present to plan for the termination process.

Within three months, the parent aide was able to close the case. Ms. G and her baby were sharing an apartment with another couple, and Ms. G found a temporary job with some potential for permanence. During working hours Ms. G's family and the foster mother cared for the baby. Ms. G was genuinely excited about the possibilities for her future and she was feeling more competent as a parent.

The final case to be described in this section has been among the most challenging of the approximately 280 cases served by the parent aide program in its first six years.

CASE 4

Ms. N. Ms. N, aged 27, was referred for a parent aide by both a drug dependency program and the Family Advocate program of the Coordinating Committee. Ms. N's son was 3 weeks old at the time of the referral and still in the hospital because Ms. N was living in a boarding house and had no place for him. Mrs. N was being seen daily at the methadone clinic and reported as experiencing considerable anxiety about meeting the needs of her infant.

The paternal grandmother offered some support to Ms. N, but her own family was not interested or involved.

The baby's father was an ex-addict, currently unemployed. Ms. N had been divorced seven years previously from a man who was physically abusive to her. There were no children from that union. At the time of referral for a Family Advocate, Ms. N had been evicted from her apartment and needed to find a place to live in order to gain the release of her son from the hospital. A Family Advocate helped her search the market and negotiate with a landlord. As soon as this was accomplished, the advocate withdrew from the case and was replaced by a parent aide due to the urgency of the situation.

The initial case conference, held shortly after the baby's birth, brought Ms. N together with the team that would provide support for her: the parent aide, the aide's supervisor, the welfare worker, and the physician and social worker from the drug dependency unit.

The case log maintained by the parent aide contains this report of the first attempted home visit:

> Went at 2:00 to Ms. N's. She wasn't there. Waited 'til 2:30. Called office and found that she had left a note saying that she had a nose bleed . . . checked with referring worker, who told me Ms. N feared her welfare check would stop if I came and snooped around, and she was reported to have her boyfriend living there and helping her—maybe that was why she invented the nose bleed.

The parent aide returned the following week at her scheduled time, again only to find no one at home. This time a call to the office provided the information that Ms. N had taken her infant to the hospital because his foot had been burned. The aide went directly to the hospital, where it was decided that the burn was accidental and that the infant would have to remain in the hospital for ten days.

During the next week the parent aide maintained telephone contact with mother, supporting her involvement in the course of treatment for her son. The parent aide located a stroller for the baby which she brought to Ms. N at the time the baby was returned home. The gift of the stroller was a statement of acceptance and caring that was positively interpreted by Ms. N and useful in the development of the relationship between the parent aide and the client.

Ms. N was faithful in maintaining her methadone appointments and her visits to her therapist, herself an ex-addict. The parent aide helped enroll Ms. N and her baby in the neighborhood health clinic and then helped her to establish Medicaid eligibility and become certified for an income supplement to upgrade the quality of her housing. The baby's health was good and the foot healed well with no further treatment indicated. The parent aide took her grocery shopping and to the laundromat regularly. As Ms. N became more trusting, she shared with the parent aide her boyfriend's hope for getting a job and staying drug free.

The parent aide modeled infant feeding for Ms. N and helped her understand the importance of adequate nutrition for both the baby and herself. She worked with her to find dishes, pots and pans, and furniture. When Ms. N moved into the apartment, she had brought with her a kitchen set and a mattress.

At the case conference held seven months after the parent aide placement, Ms. N was still maintaining her therapy and medication schedules, her boyfriend was working, and she was planning to move to a better apartment. The baby's health continued to be good, and he was well cared for. His immunizations were on schedule, and he was being seen regularly by his primary physician. Ms. N acknowledged the help of the parent aide and asked that she remain with her.

As Ms. N's self-esteem increased, she became interested in her own future; her welfare dependence concerned her, and she expressed interest in going back to school to develop a skill. As she had no mailbox, the aide suggested that the catalogues for which she had sent be mailed to the agency's address. Her education was to be negotiated with the State Department of Vocational Rehabilitation.

Mrs. N had to confront separation from her son when she became serious about schooling. This was difficult for her; she had never used a baby-sitter before and her son was 1 year old. The aide helped her to find a competent sitter and helped her to be comfortable with leaving him. The aide also was involved in suggesting some changes in the sleeping arrangements, encouraging Mrs. N to let the baby sleep in his own bed rather than with her.

The aide was a key participant at the baby's first birthday, which was celebrated at a local MacDonald's with ten children and eight adult family members. This marked a change in the relationship between Ms. N and her mother, which had been angry and painful.

While the parent aide was on vacation, she received a long letter from Ms. N in which she spoke of her lovely new apartment and said, "I'm glad you'll be coming home soon. The baby and I miss you. I don't have a living room set or dining room set yet so we won't be able to sit when you come over, but at least now I can offer you a cup of coffee from a decent kitchen in a clean cup. I used to feel rude because I didn't offer, but I was too ashamed." The letter was signed by both the baby and Ms. N.

As Ms. N became increasingly independent, her relationship with her boyfriend became strained. He was jealous of her relationship with others, resented her interests outside of the family, and often prevented her from taking part in activities which she found appealing, including participation in a public hearing on income maintenance. His anger eventually erupted, and Ms. N became the victim of abusive beatings, which drove her to the Battered Women's Shelter to protect herself and her son.

A strategy to ensure the safety of Ms. N and her baby was developed and implemented. Legal Aid helped Ms. N get a restraining order to keep her boyfriend away; the parent aide helped her to obtain other entitlements to prepare to take care of herself and her son. The aide also accompanied her to court.

At 18 months, the baby was enrolled in a nursery school early stimulation program to offer him an opportunity for socialization. Prior to acceptance in the program, he was evaluated and found to be developmentally age appropriate with some hyperactivity.

The relationship between Ms. N and her boyfriend became increasingly problematic. The boyfriend returned to live in Ms. N's apartment and returned to his drug habit, which he used all of his income to support. Ms. N continued to pursue her own career training options while attempting to deal with the chaos resulting from her domestic entanglement. Her fear for her own and her son's well-being prevented her from acting decisively. Her therapist of that time, a psychiatrist, prescribed tranquilizers to help her cope with her anxiety.

The deteriorating relationship with her boyfriend caused Ms. N to move to the Battered Women's Shelter for a second time and to seek emergency housing. Her parents helped her move and agreed to store her furniture. During this period of disruption, case-specific meetings were called monthly, and Ms. N's mother was invited to attend.

Ms. N moved from the shelter to a motel with the help of the Welfare Department and began to look for subsidized housing in other nearby communities. The parent aide assisted in finding day care providers in these towns, although the child continued in the stimulation program.

Twenty-two months after the initial referral, Ms. N was working with a family advocate to find housing once again. She had developed an eye problem and required a series of appointments with her ophthalmologist. The parent agency found a volunteer to care for her son while she received treatment.

Although it appears that little had changed in twenty-two months of work with Ms. N and her child, in fact this was not the case. Ms. N had changed in many important ways. She had slowly gained control of her life and had begun to make decisions which were in the best interests of herself and her son. She had separated from her boyfriend, sought medical care for her child and herself, and committed herself to seeking opportunities to improve the potential for both of them. She was a devoted mother; her son has responded well and was developing appropriately.

The parent aide program made a commitment to Ms. N to remain with her until her family situation was stabilized and her own network became strong enough to offer her the support she wanted and used. The outcome of this case was considered positive, but it was far from ideal. The experience of the program suggests that we lack the capability to provide the ideal environment for children in families such as those described in this section. The importance of the continuity of cultural ties, social options, and pride in one's family can make a difference in the child's mastery of other deficits, as noted by Solnit (1980). Coupled with the child's need for permanency and constancy of caregiving, these factors make persuasive arguments for supporting the natural mother–child relationship.

To be accepted by the parent on a voluntary basis, support programs must offer services that are nonjudgmental and unburdened by the values and preferences of the helpers. The only parental behaviors which should be clearly discouraged are those which fail to protect the child or meet the child's basic needs. Aides use the parent–helper relationship, their own resources, and the resources available in the community to help the family make a more useful life-style adaptation. Changes in functioning are incremental, occurring over many months. Among the goals of such intervention is the prevention of further, more serious dysfunction and the potential erosion of the family's own resources. An evaluation of federally funded child abuse and neglect projects (Hefler and Kemper, 1976) found that "Clients who received lay services (i.e., parent aides and Parents Anonymous) are the clients most likely to show improved functioning (in those areas cited as problems at intake) by the end of treatment. . . . The lay model does have the strongest effect of the service models studied" (p. xxvi).

Parent aides cannot change the patterns of family interaction in isolation. The availability of a range of community-based services is critical for families whose needs are complex and diffuse, often involving every aspect of family functioning. A successful parent aide intervention represents a meaningful collaboration between the family, the community, and the public sector. It is a collaboration from which each component benefits but none more than the children, who do not have to wait until it is too late to make the family a safe place.

Not all cases accepted for service are successful.

CASE 5

Ms. P. Ms. P is an example of a case in which the community committed itself to a massive infusion of service in order to maintain family unity and was unable to achieve its goals. Connecticut's (1980) "Standards for the Removal and the Return of Children" supported keeping the four children (ranging in age from 4 years to 3 months at the time of referral) with their mother.

Ms. P, aged 25, lived with her parents, grandparents, and siblings in a household of sixteen persons. During the three years in which the parent aide program was involved with this family, the Children's Protective Service agency, a mental health clinic, a child guidance clinic, a private pediatrician, hospital social workers, nurses, school teachers, and the Welfare Department were represented at the eleven case conferences facilitated by the supervisor. The areas initially identified as problematic for Ms. P were child management, discipline, budget, independent living, and getting a high school equivalency degree. Strategies for addressing these issues were to seek developmental evaluations of the children with transportation provided by the parent aide, define the roles of the many adult family members, register the older children in kindergarten and Head Start programs, arrange for food stamps, help her to meet her children's medical needs (one child had ophthalmologic problems, and one was subject to seizures), and enroll one child in a special educational program.

Family life was chaotic; the children were enuretic and without limits or boundaries, there were no established mealtimes, and mother provided little personal hygiene. Children were not bathed regularly and became lice infested; drug and alcohol abuse were evident.

The parent aide supervisor sought consideration from one of the multidisciplinary teams of the Coordinating Committee in an effort to plan the intervention more effectively. The preventive service worker, the parent aide, the pediatrician, and the child guidance clinic were enlisted for specific tasks. The children's protective service worker acknowledged that the state was closing the case.

At a review of the case five months later by the multidisciplinary team, it was recommended that the parent aide become the case manager and limit the scope of her work to attempt to improve Ms. P's parenting skills. A word of caution was added: if mother didn't work cooperatively, the parent aide should be terminated.

The parent aide remained with the family for two years beyond the case review. Although there were times of improved functioning, these times could not be sustained. Children were sent home from school because of the severity of their lice infestations, and they were subject to frequent respiratory infections. To ensure the children's attendance at school or camp, the parent aide visited the house at 7:00 A.M. to prepare them for the day or, occasionally, to assist mother in taking them to their medical appointments.

The parent aide assumed responsibility for making and keeping appointments for testing or developmental evaluations and kept in constant contact with Ms. P to remind her of what had been scheduled. Family assessments recommended involvement with various programs offering stimulation and learning opportunities and supported maintenance of family integrity.

At times the family found itself with no food, no electricity, and no hot water, which resulted in many infections and frequent trips to the emergency room. The children's father lived with the family intermittently. Ms. P and the children would be saddened by his precipitous disappearances and joyous upon his return. He was not able to sustain an intimate relationship over time.

With serious concern about the family's functioning, Protective Services reopened the case and entered into an agreement with Ms. P requiring her to get the older children to school or to summer camp every morning, bring the youngest child's immunizations up to date, save $50 monthly for her own apartment, consider reapplying for subsidized housing, and protect her children from other family members who might hurt them. Protective Services agreed to assist with housing, provide support, and arrange for voluntary placement if it seemed desirable. Recognizing the chaotic home environment, Ms. P made an attempt to live with an aunt in a more structured environment, but even with the encouragement of the parent aide, she could not separate from her family and quickly returned home.

Ms. P's ability to protect her children from injury or keep them from antisocial acts became major issues which the parent aide repeatedly attempted to address. This was further complicated when Ms. P became depressed following the sudden death of a male sibling and developed a sleep disorder. She was less able to meet the needs of her children. At this point, the parent aide supervisor, the parent aide, and Ms. P met together and mutually agreed to termination of the aide's placement. For three years the community offered this family a wide range of support. Mental health, medical, and educational resources were used but not truly useful because Ms. P was unable to organize herself or her family. Competent helpers felt frustrated and helpless working with the extended family. They were constrained by the limits of their own ability to meet the needs of this family and did not know how best to intervene.

The failure of the agency and the community to help Ms. P and improve the prognosis for her children points up the need for careful study. In what types of cases can parent aides be most effective? At what point can we say we have stretched ourselves as far as we know how, and, in the best interests of the child, we can no longer work to maintain family integrity? Who should make this decision?

Cases such as Ms. P's present a serious challenge; for her children the attempts to intervene in their lives, which were thought to be in their best interests, may have had negative consequences. Had no support been given to the family, its disintegration might have accelerated more rapidly and in turn led more quickly to placement in a safe and nurturing home. This is the dilemma that sometimes confronts us and for which we have no easy answers. As

Rutter (1972) has advised, it is important that we do not oversell our capacity to achieve change in family functioning. However, the number of cases in which parent aides have been useful in marshaling resources and assisting families to nurture more effectively exceed, by a ratio of approximately 3:1, the number of cases in which little progress has been made toward treatment goals.

Further study is needed to determine if certain indicators exist which could suggest families who may effectively use community support programs, as well as those who should be screened out at the time of intake. As we experiment with interventions, time can run out for the children we are trying to serve. Greater understanding of the extents and limitations of parent aide programs will help to utilize this potentially helpful intervention more effectively.

Teaching Homemaker

Expanding its role in the community, the parent agency entered into a collaboration with a local school system and a nursing program to attempt to prevent adolescent pregnancies and to provide assistance and support to adolescent parents. The program components included a school-based education program on family life and human sexuality for students in grades 7, 8, and 9, direct services to pregnant students and student parents in the school system, and direct services to school-age parents not enrolled in school.

The objectives of the program designed for pregnant students and parenting students in the school system included the provision of a parent education curriculum to foster healthy parent–child relationships, prevent undesirable repeat pregnancies, promote adolescent development, encourage the enrollment of all pregnant teens in WIC programs, and increase the rate of teenage pregnant patients registering for prenatal care in their first trimester.

The objectives of the program designed for school-age parents who had dropped out of school were to link this group with existing educational, health, and day care services for the purpose of helping them to complete their education, postpone or prevent a second pregnancy, involve the teenage father with his new family, teach mothers effective parenting by providing support and instruction within their own homes, facilitate a peer support group, and teach daily living skills.

The teaching homemaker program was to provide in-home and peer support for teenage mothers. Initially designed to be time-limited and to differ from the parent aide program in the duration of the intervention, in fact, the teaching homemaker remained with families for longer than the eight sessions initially intended to constitute the service.

Prior to the implementation of the program, the agency staff developed a project guide to assist the teaching homemaker in the role of parent educator. Teaching parenting skills; identifying community resources, appropriate and affordable living arrangements; teaching daily living skills; supporting mother's return to school; job training and job searching; and reducing isolation were identified as the general topic areas for work with teenage mothers. As a voluntary program in which mothers' preferences were paramount, the teaching homemaker took into account the mother's own wishes and cultural patterns regarding child rearing.

The teaching homemaker modeled a range of mother–child interactions, including hugging, touching, story-telling, disciplining, and praising. She assisted the parent to support her child's cognitive development by teaching mothers appropriate language use with the baby, suggesting safe ways for eventual exploration of the environment, and preparing mothers to accept infant and toddler behavior.

To help the young mother cope with economic reality, the teaching homemaker reviewed tenant responsibilities for paying rent, utilities, and security deposits, as well as the designation of responsibilities for repairs, care, and upkeep. The teaching homemaker was able to assist with money management and budgeting, grocery shopping, menu planning, and nutrition. The homemaker was able to accompany the teenage mother to appointments and special activities, and to help her identify and utilize those community resources which were relevant and potentially useful.

Case Studies

Case profiles taken from the records of the teaching homemaker project describe two of the families served in the first year of the program.

CASE 1

Jennie was a pregnant 18-year-old when she was referred to the teaching homemaker program by the Protective Services agency. She did not have the support of an adult member of an extended family, had considerable anxiety about her ability to parent, and was in need of health, social, and educational services.

Jennie's first visit with the teaching homemaker and the program supervisor took place the month prior to delivery. The first session which followed this interview lasted three hours. The teaching homemaker took Jennie shopping for the new baby and made plans to meet with her again shortly to help her choose the things she wanted to take with her to the hospital when the baby was born.

Jennie and the teaching homemaker met for a total of twenty-two sessions before termination took place; each session lasted approximately three hours, comparable to a parent aide visit. The issues which were prominent in these sessions were fears about childbirth, expectations of motherhood, and the type of mother Jennie wanted to be. The teaching homemaker accompanied Jennie on a visit to the hospital to familiarize her with the surroundings prior to delivery, and after delivery, took her to the Welfare Office, where she claimed entitlements on behalf of her baby.

The teaching homemaker helped Jennie enter a school-based program for young mothers, which she attended with her child, and was instrumental in finding a tutor to prepare her to take the high school equivalency examination. Finally, she and her son were enrolled in an infant–toddler play group, where she was helped to further develop her parenting skills in a supportive environment.

CASE 2

Phyllis was a 17-year-old mother of two children; her daughter was 2 years old, and her son was one. Phyllis was referred to the program by the school system because she was in danger of losing her status as a high school sophomore. She was approaching the twenty-day limit for absences and had a record of excessive tardiness. Working with Phyllis, the teaching homemaker learned that her absences were due to some major changes in her living arrangements. During the past school term, Phyllis had decided to move into a rented room with her two children, leaving the foster mother with whom she had lived since infancy. She found the transition to independent living difficult; she had trouble coping with being an adolescent mother and a student. Although she discussed her health problems with the teaching homemaker, she was unpredictable in keeping her medical appointments. She was warm and accepting of the teaching homemaker, but establishing a daily routine, finding appropriate day care, and moving to more appropriate housing were all areas to be addressed with the homemaker and resolved before Phyllis could maintain her educational plan.

A major difficulty encountered in the effort to serve adolescent mothers was the shortage of acceptable low-income housing. For the adolescent who feels, as Phyllis did, that she wants or must make a home of her own, there is virtually no housing available.

Furthermore, women under the age of 18 are unable to enter into legally binding contracts, which makes signing a lease an impossibility. The agency attempted to find some housing for young mothers and their children through an intergenerational home sharing project but found that older persons are reluctant to have young mothers and their children come to live with them. Recruiting families willing to share their homes with teenage mothers and their children through a foster care network may offer a possible alternative. It may be easier for a potential foster family to accept a child and a teenage mother than it is for an elderly home provider to accept a home sharer who brings a young infant with her. In such a program the teenage mother might provide care for her own child and pay rent and/or exchange service. In return, she would have a safe place to live and the possibility of the social support of the foster family. A teaching homemaker could be available to both teen mother and foster mother.

Parent aides and teaching homemakers were concerned primarily with intrafamilial relationships. They served families in their own homes and were encouraged to develop long-term, trusting relationships designed to encourage sharing, increase self-confidence, and improve the quality of family life. The presumption underlying these programs was that family functioning is dependent upon parental attitudes, feelings, and relationships. However, families do not exist apart from the larger society; they are influenced by environmental forces which impact upon them. Poverty, social isolation, lack of housing, unemployment, and cutbacks in entitlement programs are stressors which can overwhelm already fragile families and threaten family integrity.

In 1984, the Family Support Service (FSS) was added to the In-Home Service programs of the Coordinating Council. A collaboration between DCYS, the Coordinating Council, and the Yale Child Study Center, FSS was offered to families whose children were identified as in imminent need of placement. The Family Support Service team included a DCYS intake worker, a parent aide, and a clinician who intervened in order to prevent placement. Assessment and treatment planning took place within the home, utilizing the skills of the team members. FSS staff remained with the family for approximately twelve weeks; when necessary, the case was transferred to appropriate community resources for long-term involvement.

The Coordinating Council for Children in Crisis is no longer a part of the Family Services Collaboration. The Family Support Service at Yale Child Study Center has been expanded to include the original FSS program, now known as the Intensive Family Intervention Program. It continues to provide intensive, time-limited in-home service to children referred by DCYS because of imminent risk of out-of-home placement due to abuse, neglect, or abandonment. Similar programs, which also use a team consisting of a family support worker and a clinician, serve children at risk of placement because of HIV infection or maternal drug use. Additional programs are being considered for children of mentally ill parents and parents involved with the criminal justice system. The Coordinating Council for Children in Crisis continues to provide parent aide and family advocate services in the region and is an important postdischarge resource for families served by the Family Support Service. Programs similar to the one described in this chapter have been replicated throughout Connecticut.

Case Management and Advocacy

The case management and advocacy component of the Coordinating Council presumes that families are profoundly influenced by external as well as internal stressors. Environmental or ecological problems can contribute to family breakdown. It is not unusual, for example, for workers to suggest that children be placed because a family cannot locate a suitable home or because a landlord threatens eviction and the family sees no alternative to placement.

In accordance with the mission and assumptions of the Coordinating Council, the Family Advocate program was conceived as a means of providing assistance and empowering client families to deal with environmental problems. The program reflects Kenniston's assumption that improving environmental conditions will result in improved mental and physical health (Kenniston and the Carnegie Council, 1977). Advocates worked directly with families referred to the program by other professionals, helping them deal with housing problems by applying for Section Eight supplemental rent subsidies such as the Section Eight program of the Federal Housing and Urban Development (HUD) administration; forestalling evictions; providing landlord lists; suggesting possible home-sharing arrangements; and teaching good landlord–tenant relations. Advocates negotiated with utility companies on the client's behalf and accompanied clients to meetings and appointments where the advocate provided support and represented the interests of the family. Advocates frequently functioned as case managers, coordinating a variety of resources on the client's behalf; at all times, however, the client remained the primary decision maker. The advocate was encouraged to meet the client in the home shortly following case assignment, although much of the actual work was done by telephone. The home visit gave the advocate an opportunity to see the family in a setting in which the parent was more comfortable and at ease. The visit allowed the advocate the opportunity to gain a better understanding of the circumstances of the family's life, which could be useful in attempting to negotiate on behalf of family members.

The advocate program made use of community organizing skills, as well as the skills of a traditional case worker. Tenant organizing efforts and attempts to encourage creative market solutions to serious housing problems emerged from the program with tangible benefits for families, clients, and staff members. Systems advocacy also emerged as a necessary adjunct to the work of the program. All cases referred to the advocate program involved families with children who are considered at risk. Inadequate (for example, rat-infested) housing poses a serious threat to family health and well-being, as does a lack of refrigeration or the loss of entitlements. Adults, living in situations in which they can take no pride and which degrade and devalue them, feel undermined and inadequate as parents as well. The resulting anger and frustration may be imparted to their children, perpetuating feelings of hopelessness and despair.

It was the goal of the Family Advocate program to intervene positively in a task-oriented manner, and to increase the parents' sense of accomplishments and self-esteem in dealing with systems that were potentially threatening and antagonistic. The intervention was designed to

be short term. However, in some families a personal relationship developed, and the advocate became a continuing
source of support and encouragement, a person on the
other end of the telephone, someone to call upon when a
crisis occurred or a new problem arose. All cases were
closed with the consent of the parent and could be reopened at any time at the parent's request. The comprehensive approach inherent in the Family Advocate program reflected the findings of the Lower East Side Family
Union, Inc. (1976). Reducing stress in dysfunctional families required a willingness to become involved in all aspects
of the life of the family.

The Family Advocate program served 176 families
with 327 children during one program year; 71 percent of
the families were referred for housing problems, including
evictions, homelessless, substandard living conditions, and
landlord–tenant problems.

Assistance in claiming income maintenance or supplemental awards was the primary reason for referral in 11
percent of the cases; problems involving utilities, including
shut-offs, accounted for 8 percent; service linkage was requested for 6 percent of the families; and financial management was needed in the remaining 4 percent.

The following case studies were chosen for inclusion
in this chapter because in each case there was an infant
or young child at risk. The cases illustrate the parents'
difficulties in coping with environmental problems. The
intervention of the family advocate may have prevented
the need for more drastic remedies.

Case Studies

CASE 1

Ms. J, Ms. J, aged 23, was referred to the Family Advocate program by the Women's Clinic of the local hospital.

Ms. J had a 30-month-old daughter and was pregnant with her second child, who was due within several weeks. At the time of the referral, she was in the hospital for treatment of complications resulting from her pregnancy.

Ms. J had lost her job and her medical benefits, had no source of income, and had received two eviction notices from her current landlord. The advocate made her initial visit at the hospital and attempted to clarify the client's financial status. Ms. J already had applied for welfare and WIC for the expected baby. However, she had not heard from the welfare worker who had promised to visit Ms. J at the hospital. The advocate discovered that Ms. J's eviction was being negotiated by Ms. J's attorney and the landlord's attorney, but few details were being communicated to the client.

With Ms. J's permission, the advocate made contact with Ms. J's attorney, who welcomed her involvement; the landlord's attorney refused to talk with her. Ms. J's rent was $300 per month, and she was in arrears for four months. Negotiations were postponed until Ms. J had something with which to bargain.

Next, the advocate contacted the income maintenance office to inquire about what was happening to Ms. J's application. She was told that Ms. J needed a letter from her doctor confirming her illness and that rent payments would be covered from the date of the completed application for benefits.

The advocate made a total of eight telephone calls to collateral agencies during the day following the initial visit to the hospital. By the end of the day, the Welfare Department had decided that a visit to the client was unnecessary, and the application for income support was activated. The attorneys agreed to negotiate if Ms. J could raise some money and would consent to a schedule for rent that would include a $1200 rent repayment.

Two days later Ms. J delivered a healthy baby boy. By that time her aunt had agreed to contribute $200 toward her overdue rent. On the following work day the advocate went to the Housing Court on behalf of Ms. J, informing the judge that Ms. J had delivered her child and was attempting to raise some money to reduce her debt to the landlord. The landlord's attorney agreed to a continuance of one week if money would be forthcoming. The attorneys and the advocate agreed to meet again one week later.

A call to the hospital social worker informed the advocate that Ms. J and her baby would be discharged the following day. Her aunt had readied the apartment for their return. The advocate informed Ms. J that the income maintenance office needed the baby's birth certificate to grant an income award for him. While awaiting the start of AFDC payments to Ms. J, the advocate contacted the city welfare department as an interim income source. Several days after she returned home, Ms. J was approved for city welfare and given a $50 voucher.

The advocate contacted the landlord's attorney and found that he would accept a use-and-occupancy agreement but not a renewed lease until Ms. J paid her debt in full. With this information, the advocate was able to help negotiate a settlement in which Ms. J agreed to a case settlement of $300 to repay her debt over time by adding a monthly surcharge of $100 and to pay court and legal fees of $150. Under these conditions, her apartment was secured for fifteen months.

Once the acute housing problems were addressed, the advocate was able to concentrate on helping Ms. J with her new baby. The advocate solicited a layette for the baby from a local organization, took Ms. J to apply for food stamps, and helped her prepare a budget sheet to maximize her food stamp allocation.

Ms. J's limited budget did not stretch to cover back utility bills, and before long, her telephone was disconnected. The advocate acted as an intermediary between

Ms. J and the telephone company, eventually negotiating a limited service agreement, which reduced Ms. J's monthly costs.

Similar problems developed with other utilities, all of which required the advocate to negotiate payments in order to avert shut-offs. Contacts were made with the energy assistance program, which was able to offer additional financial aid.

With living arrangements somewhat settled, Ms. J wanted to go back to work in order to offer her children a more financially secure future. In the meantime, they were together as a family, some of the crises had been resolved, and an advocate was only a telephone call away.

CASE 2

Ms. C. Ms. C, aged 23, was the mother of two children, ages 18 months and 5 years. She was referred to the family advocate by a Head Start program. She and her children needed a place to live. She had moved into her mother's apartment in a housing project, jeopardizing her mother's rent status. If she stayed in the apartment, she and her mother would face eviction.

The advocate met with Ms. C to consider the possible alternatives available, to discuss the possibility of furniture storage, and to help her apply to the Housing Authority. When attempts to help Ms. C remain with her mother in the project were unsuccessful, the advocate decided to convene a case specific meeting to coordinate the agencies involved with the family. Representatives of the State Welfare Department, city welfare, Head Start, and the city's family relocation office reviewed the needs of the family and accepted individual assignments as part of a case plan which recognized and endorsed Ms. C's wish to remain with her mother, who provided considerable support for herself and her children.

Contacts were made with Section Eight, local realty companies, and housing project officers. The advocate and the client visited apartments and explored the possibility of her staying with extended family members. Within three months of the case specific meeting, Ms. C rented a three-bedroom apartment. Understanding the needs of the family, the housing project had not evicted them prior to their locating another apartment, and the move was orderly and unstressful. Most important, the children and family were able to remain together without interruption.

CASE 3

Ms. S. Ms. S, aged 24, lived with her 24-month-old son in a two-room apartment in the city. She was referred to the program by a social worker at a rehabilitation center, where her son was treated for a hearing impairment and for problems involving his motor coordination. She was an isolated, shy woman, with no family support and with little confidence in her ability to care for her child.

The task of managing money became the focus of the advocate's work with Ms. S, who needed to learn how to shop for food, clothing, and other essentials. The advocate taught her to look for sales; to refrain from buying convenience foods, which generally are more expensive than fresh foods; to car pool to avoid bus and taxi fares; and to use her entitlements to the best advantage. Appreciating the disproportionate amount of her grant going toward her rent, Ms. S began to look for less expensive housing. With the assistance of the advocate, she applied for a two-bedroom apartment in a new, subsidized housing project.

Both the advocate and the social worker at the Rehabilitation Center observed carefully the quality of parent–child relationship. When they were with mother, they attempted to model patterns of interaction and noticed that the child became more responsive and alert. Recognizing that Ms. S could make good use of support and encouragement, the advocate suggested to Ms. S that she might enjoy the ongoing support of a parent aide. Ms. S was enthusiastic, an intra-agency referral was made, and the advocate introduced Ms. S to the parent aide supervisor. When the advocate closed the case, Ms. S was looking forward to the placement of an aide and to the move to a larger but more affordable new apartment.

As illustrated, the advocate program was reality oriented; it generally was not possible to find ideal solutions to the problems which faced its clients. Economic constraints, insufficient community resources, societal attitudes, and national, state, and local policies, as well as personal limitations and individual capacities, had considerable influence over possible outcomes. Not all families were able to accept assistance; some demanded immediate gratification. Many had learned to distrust service providers or to "manipulate" the system for survival, but without gaining substantial, long-term benefits for themselves. At times, clients did not recognize that the failure of programs to meet their needs was often due to the professionals' lack of knowledge or society's lack of commitment; they internalized the failure and considered themselves more inadequate as a result.

The advocates themselves became angry and frustrated by the large number of housing referrals and other equally difficult requests. They felt helpless and inadequate themselves, knowing that there was little or nothing they could do to create housing opportunities when none existed or to meet other needs that defied solutions. They also became angry at those clients who they felt failed to take some responsibility for their own problems and did not follow through, all of which created a need to support staff members and provide opportunities for reviewing the agencies' methods, strategies, and goals.

Of all the agency's programs, none points up more the need to integrate services, coordinate resources, and reconsider our national policies and priorities than the work of the family advocates. Without systems change, there is little hope that the issues raised by this program will be effectively resolved; meeting the needs of children requires the involvement of every sector of our society.

Multidisciplinary Teams

The first services offered to the community by the Coordinating Council was a multidisciplinary team, facilitated by the agency director, whose members were drawn from the agency board. A child psychiatrist, pediatrician, social worker, attorney, and a nonprofessional child advocate volunteered to meet monthly as a group to provide consultation to other professionals in the formulation of treatment plans, identification of appropriate resources, and resolution of disputes and conflicts. The team was designed to enhance cooperation between public and private agencies by stressing the need for collaboration between agencies, involving persons working in a wide range of community services as team members, and inviting persons specific to the case referred for consultation to participate in case presentations and discussions.

Of available teams, two teams could be used by any agency in the community; one team met with the intake unit of the regional DCYS office. Families were not invited to the meeting; the meetings were solely for the use of the professional community and provided an opportunity to question, debate, reach consensus, and identify resources. Although supported financially and conceptually by the DCYS management, not all protective services workers were comfortable using teams. Initially, some workers found the experience stressful, feeling called upon to defend past actions, rather than to address the unmet needs

of the child and the family. The teams were most successful when the team members and community workers focused upon the task of considering the best interests of
the child, identifying appropriate resources to meet those
needs, and deciding upon the most effective roles for those
who would remain involved with the family. Referrals
came from a range of community agencies, including
DCYS, preventive services, local hospitals, schools, child
guidance clinics, and day care programs. Largely because
of the dedication and commitment of team members,
teams became the effective means of providing expert assistance to agencies and institutions whose budgets did not
include funding for professional consultation.

An illustrative case was referred to the team by a preventive services worker. It involved a maternal grandmother, her 16-year-old daughter, four grandchildren
ranging in age from 8 to 1 year for whom she was the
primary caretaker, and the mother of the children, who
had a history of chronic psychiatric problems, with frequent hospitalizations. The case specific people included
the family advocate from the Coordinating Council, the
DCYS worker and supervisor, and representatives of the
City Housing Authority. The team considered the many
services which were needed by the grandmother in order
for her to continue to provide a home for herself, her
grandchildren, and her daughter. Agreements were made
which included designating the family advocate as case
manager, gaining the promise of the housing authority to
find the grandmother a larger apartment with an appropriate lease, offering assistance in financial planning, and
identifying additional income sources. The goal of the intervention was to prevent any further disruption for the
children, stabilize the family, and ensure the continuity
of the children's caretaking. The possibility of a transfer
guardianship would eventually be discussed by DCYS with

grandmother and mother. Although all participants appeared to be satisfied with the progress made at the team
meeting, a review was scheduled in a month's time to assess
the success of the plan.

It is the type of collaboration which this case illustrates, often on a level of concrete service provision, which
not only works in the interest of the specific child and
family presented for discussion, but also helps to build
trusting professional relationships which may smooth the
way toward better services for other families as well.

HOME SHARING SERVICES

The Coordinating Council, in an attempt to meet the
pressing need of young mothers and their children for
safe, low-cost housing, created an intergenerational home
sharing program in collaboration with the regional Agency
on Aging. This program attempted to match young mothers and their children with elderly persons living alone
and in need of someone with whom to share expenses and/
or the household responsibilities. Program staff interviewed, screened, recommended matches, and provided
follow-up for program participants. Funded initially by
a local foundation, the program made matches between
sixteen elderly persons and sixteen young mothers in two
years. The program had been considerably more successful in matching elderly persons with single adults, who
are more likely to meet the needs and expectations of the
homeowner.

To meet the goal of the Coordinating Council to serve
the needs of young mothers and children more closely,
the agency added a new dimension to the home sharing
program, now seeking to recruit homeowners from a pool
of people who wished to become foster parents but had
not yet been licensed. They were thought to be more likely
than elderly homeowners to accept a young child into their

home and welcome the addition of the caretaking young mother who was able to pay rent and assume responsibility for the needs of her child. Both the young mother and her child would receive support from the foster parents, who could help teach parenting skills while reducing the social isolation of both the mother and her child.

CASE ILLUSTRATION

Ms. C. Ms. C was a 20-year-old mother with a 2-year-old child. After the birth of her child, mother lived with her own mother and father until her father's alcoholism created a potentially dangerous environment in which the child was at risk of physical abuse. Although Ms. C was under pressure not to leave her parents, she decided to seek a way to provide a more stable home. Project Home Share was able to match Ms. C with a family that had sought to become foster parents but were found ineligible because the available bedroom and bathroom in their home were not on the same floor as the master bedroom, and thus not in compliance with a licensing requirement. Ms. C and her child were able to enjoy the privacy of a room on the second floor with no risk that the child would be unattended.

Ms. C and her child became part of the match family. Mr. D, the homeowner, had a disability which kept him home and would enable him to provide child care if Ms. C decided to get a job, something she was considering. Ms. C paid her share of the rent from her AFDC check and helped with some household chores.

When the D family goes to watch their 14-year-old son play basketball, Ms. C and her child go along. They eat, shop, and watch television as a family. The match has had positive consequences for two families, each of which has benefited from the relationship.

Project staff, who interviewed, screened, and introduced the families, remain involved on a continuing basis to offer support and assistance.

The programs of support for families described in this chapter represent some of the many services which we believe can be useful to families at certain critical times in their development. Families with few supports of their own, stressed by the demands of young children and by poverty, isolation, and lack of education, and deprived of self-respect and dignity, can be helped to stabilize and to function more effectively with access to voluntary, community-based service that offers support, understanding, acceptance, and assistance.

The experiences of the Coordinating Council, although not yet systematically researched, suggest that reaching out to families before they are fixed in patterns of dysfunctional interactions can be effective. Modeling behaviors, creating opportunities for success, and empowering families who have felt themselves to be powerless are some of the primary tasks of support programs. When parents are allowed to be in control, to make decisions about their own lives and those of their children, to terminate the service at will, and to request resumption when it seems appropriate and useful to them, they will gain a sense of accomplishment and ego strength which will inform other behaviors and will enhance their ability to parent effectively. It is almost never too early to offer such support to families effectively, but for many children and families it is often too late.

References

Connecticut (1980), Standards for the removal and return of children by the Department of Children and Youth Services. In: *Protective Services Manual*, Vol. 2. Hartford, CT: Connecticut Department of Children and Youth Services.

Helfer, R., & Kempe, C., Eds. (1968), *The Battered Child*. Chicago: University of Chicago Press.

———— (1976), *Child Abuse and Neglect, the Family and the Community.* Cambridge, MA: Ballinger Publishing Co.

Kenniston K., & the Carnegie Council (1977), *All Our Children.* New York & London: Harcourt, Brace & Jovanovich.

Lower East Side Family Union (1976), *Annual Report.* New York: Lower East Side Family Union.

National Center for Comprehensive Emergency Services to Children (NCCESC) (1976), *Community Guide*, 2nd ed. Nashville, TN: NCCESC.

Rutter, M. (1972), Prevention of children's psychosocial disorders: Myth and substance. *Pediatrics*, 70:883–894.

Solnit, A. J. (1980), Too much reporting, too little service: Roots and prevention of child abuse. In: *Child Abuse, an Agenda for Action*, ed. G. Gerbner, C. Ross, & E. Zigler. New York: Oxford University Press.

U.S. Department of Health, Education and Welfare—National Center for Health Services Research (1974), *Evaluation of Child Abuse and Neglect Demonstration Projects, 1974–1977*, Vols. 1 & 2. DHEW Publication No. (PHS) 79-3217-1, p. xxvi. Washington, DC: DHEW.

Young-Saxon, M. (1983), Working with paraprofessionals. Typescript.

Part III:
Clinical Responses to Infants, Toddlers, and Parents in Troubled Relationships

Addressing distortions, conflicts, and near derailments in the relationships between and among very young children and their parents is, in many ways, the core of infant–family practice. Yet as the three case reports in this section illustrate, it is by no means a simple business for parents to get timely and appropriate help in supporting the development of their infants, and themselves, during the earliest years of life. When parents and practitioners *are* able to take preventive measures, however, the resulting developmental gains can be extraordinarily gratifying for all concerned.

The chapters by Shonkoff and Brazelton, Jeree Pawl, and Roth and Morrison describe infants, toddlers, and families who would not, when we encounter them, fit criteria of "risk" that frequently control access to developmental services. But all three families are in pain, and without help from outside the family, the development of the infants is likely to be compromised. In Shonkoff and Brazelton's report, the parents gained access to a multidisciplinary child development service because of their ability to verbalize their distress at 7-month-old Suzanna's sleep problem, which was an exhausting indicator of their difficulty in adjusting to their new and long-deferred roles as parents. Mr. and Mrs. Lopez and Bonita, aged 2½, were referred to Pawl's program by the pediatrician at a city–county hospital because of Bonita's behavior problems, which concerned the doctor and were affirmed by her mother as a great trial and worry. The self-referred Jordans, described by Roth and Morrison, called about their toddler Bobby, who was their ticket of admission to a service in which they could work on their marital problems. In each instance, the family situation was such that the development of the child and the family's health were already compromised and in danger of further difficulty.

A Conceptual Framework

Whatever immediate problem or symptom brings a family with an infant to their attention, the clinicians whose work is reported in the following chapters look to the family as a whole, as well as to each of its individual members, for help in understanding the meaning of the current pain. Viewing the family as an evolving system, upon which the birth and early development of a child inevitably have a major impact, helps the practitioner to put presenting problems in context and to focus on strengthening ongoing relationships. The family as a dynamic system is understood to be more complex than the characteristics of its individual members. At the same time, attention to each parent's unique personal history and cultural context, as well as to the individuality of each child, prevents the clinician from making oversimplified formulations of patterns of family functioning. The adaptations and adjustments that must be singly and mutually accomplished by father, mother, and child are implicit in the approach.

Responsiveness to the Individual Needs of a Particular Child and Family

As the following three case reports illustrate (and as the preceding chapters in this volume also emphasize), a thorough, thoughtful assessment of the child and family's situation is essential to an individualized clinical response. It is also important to recognize that assessment is itself *part* of a clinical response, not simply a prelude to intervention. And while, depending on the clinical setting, the initial assessment of a child and family may take place during a single morning or over a number of weeks, assessment must always be a continuing process.

Shonkoff and Brazelton, Pawl, and Roth and Morrison describe their assessment processes in some detail. Each clinical setting uses a mix of developmental testing protocols and observation of play and parent–infant interaction. In addition, each writer emphasizes specific assessment approaches that he or she finds particularly important.

Brazelton, a pediatrician, performs a physical examination of the baby in the course of his first visit with a child and family. He notes that "In the course of the physical, I can usually tell a certain amount about social reaction, stranger anxiety, how both baby and parents handle stress. As a pediatrician, I find the physical exam is a paradigm so familiar that I can assess the child and parent's reactions all the time I am examining the child. Any individual difference in either child's or parent's behavior sets off a signal for me" (p. 187).

Pawl and her colleagues at the Infant–Parent Program of San Francisco General Hospital conduct initial assessments consisting of four or five home visits and one office visit during as many weeks. Pawl emphasizes that the assessment process is designed to evaluate not only the child's affective, social, and cognitive functioning and the quality of the parents' caregiving practices but also the parents' willingness to accept intervention and their ability to use it on behalf of the baby.

The Parent–Infant Development Service at the University of Chicago, described by Roth and Morrison:

> [T]ypically conduct[s] comprehensive diagnostic evaluations that include medical examinations; neuropsychological assessments of infant functioning and temperament; evaluation of parenting functioning and parenting capabilities; evaluation of infant play; evaluation of parent–infant

and family–infant interactions; and evaluation of the family's environment, living conditions, and social supports as perceived by the parents [p. 232].

The initial diagnostic profile of the infant–family unit that is developed as a result of this extensive evaluation is used by staff to determine "who participates in the treatment ('the strategy'), what the target of treatment should be to begin with, and what the emphasis of the treatment should be" (p. 233). The use of formal ratings on the PIDS' Infant–Family Assessment Profile enables staff to document the functioning of all family members across many areas, and to chart gains made during the course of intervention.

The Helping Relationship

The helping relationship in each of these reports, while different as to duration, style, setting, and emphasis on certain of its elements, is characterized by mutual respect and a therapeutic alliance. The role of the interventionist is that of interpreter of the child to the parents, translator of behavioral communications from child to parent, and at times mediator between them. The interventionist may also offer interpretations of the adults' feelings and attitudes, when timely and appropriate.

Brazelton and Shonkoff illustrate how the pediatric setting and procedures can yield a rich store of information about interactions and feelings which opens the door to addressing a specific issue, conceptualized in this case as an issue of separation. Recommendations about management are offered, but not until there has been an exploration of factors important in the family's distress. The perceptiveness of a psychologically sophisticated pediatrician, the timing of his advice, the parents' readiness for help, and their increasing trust in their consultant and then in themselves, are evident in this short-term treatment.

In Pawl's case the efficient and rich context of home visiting for diagnosis and therapeutic work is illustrated. The family's daily existence and their experience with one another quickly come to attention and are combined with visits to the office for other aspects of assessment. Developmental guidance is identified as the primary mode of intervention in this case after an initial assessment that included consideration of the degree to which emotional support, concrete assistance, developmental guidance, or more introspective types of therapy were needed. In this case the relatively brief and intensive intervention was directed toward helping the parents understand and respond appropriately to Bonita's behavior. Situational factors in the life of the family and not the parents' "ghosts" were responsible for their distress. Improvements in the child's behavior during the course of therapy facilitated her parents' ability to see her as an essentially normal, attractive child, and further modified their own attitudes and behavior toward her. The improved quality of their interactions with Bonita and with one another both manifested and enhanced a positive developmental process. The family's ability to come to trust and use the therapist as guide and as an enabler in locating other services they needed and wanted represented another accomplishment achieved through the helping relationship.

Roth and Morrison present the 17-month-long treatment of Mr. and Mrs. Jordan and Bobby, describing in detail the particular aspects of psychodynamic and systems theory that guided them in the treatment of this family. In particular, the recognition and clarification of tranference manifestations and the empathic reflection of them are emphasized as an important dynamic in the healing process.

In the interaction with Bobby, the therapist's response to his verbal and nonverbal communications illustrates the process of observing and conveying the meaning of the child's experience to the parents and the parents' experience to the child.

It is worth noting the strong involvement of fathers in all three of the therapeutic relationships described in this section. While one hopes that the involvement of both parents in efforts to support the development of young children will soon be the norm, this is by no means currently the case. Shonkoff and Brazelton, Pawl, and Roth and Morrison offer valuable insights about the eagerness of fathers from all cultural backgrounds to be full participants in their children's lives. These reports also suggest ways in which clinicians can support the involvement of fathers in both the therapeutic process and the daily lives of families.

The System of Care

Each of the chapters in this section reports a successful entry into the mental health system either through an appropriate referral or through the family's own initiative. For each such well-served case there are many others who are denied appropriate care because there is no resource, because the family cannot afford services or is ineligible for free care, because services are not delivered when they would have the most impact, or because practitioners lack necessary skills.

A great deal of thought is being given to how to make emotional support widely available to families of infants and toddlers. Community-based family resource programs, home visiting initiatives that reach out to all new parents, prompt response to families in crisis, and more culturally sensitive service delivery are all possible approaches. As such initiatives are planned, it is important to keep in mind the qualifications of the people who will be working with infants, toddlers, and their families and the way in which mental health concepts can become embedded in all infant–family services. The reports of Shonkoff and Brazelton, Pawl, and Roth and Morrison illustrate these issues well. Sleep disturbances in infancy, separation fears in toddlerhood, and troubled relationships between parents are "ordinary" problems, but a great deal of skill may be necessary to assist in their resolution. Expanding the number of skilled people available to support families with infants and toddlers is a major challenge to the field. One would hope, for example, that an increasing emphasis on developmental and family issues in the training of primary health care providers would enable many practitioners to be sensitive to the family issues behind sleep disturbances such as Suzanna's (although it will probably always be the case that certain families will value only contact with "specialists"). One would hope that as our country becomes more culturally diverse, we will find ways to surmount language barriers that keep primary care providers ignorant of the family's background or current life, as was the case initially with Bonita and her family. We must also be careful that enthusiasm for a particular treatment approach, such as home visiting, does not discount the importance of highly competent practitioners. The skilled and sensitive intervention described by Pawl and by Roth and Morrison cannot be expected of an untrained "friendly visitor." While community workers have important roles to play in supporting families, their responsibilities must be commensurate with their skills and the supervision available to them.

It is also important to acknowledge the role of university-affiliated centers of excellence in fostering competent practice with infants, toddlers, and their families. Settings such as the ones described by Shonkoff and Brazelton, Pawl, and Roth and Morrison train scores of professionals from a wide range of disciplines, who can then bring their clinical and supervisory expertise to communities across the country.

5

Paradise Lost—Delayed Parenthood in the Carefully Planned Life

Jack P. Shonkoff, M.D., T. Berry Brazelton, M.D.

The case study of Suzanna and her parents is rich in the fundamental developmental issues of the earliest years of life: the process of separation–individuation, the effects of the first child on the marital relationship, and the management of a common developmental–behavioral concern, such as sleep disturbance. The case study is also embedded in the social context of deferred childbearing among professional couples, a growing but poorly studied phenomenon in American society. Dr. Brazelton was the clinician in the case; Dr. Shonkoff was primary author of the discussion.

Dr. and Mrs. C brought their 7-month-old daughter Suzanna to the Child Development Unit of the Children's Hospital in Boston. They had sought advice and support from their family pediatrician about her sleep problems, and from a second doctor to whom he referred them. Mrs. C called me (TBB) in desperation one morning and I referred her to our multidisciplinary clinic at Children's Hospital, which has a pediatrician, a nurse, child development observers, a social worker, and a child psychiatrist.

At the clinic, team members observe the family in the diagnostic phase through a one-way screen as the family is interviewed by the pediatrician or nurse who is in charge of their case. The child's temperament, responses to stress, and developmental level are a major part of the diagnostic assessment. As the family and the interviewer reach an understanding of the nature of the problem, the family is given an opportunity to "break for coffee." The interviewer consults the observers. By this time, the child has been observed in a play and diagnostic test situation—either with the parents or in the playroom. Plans for management of the case are considered by the interviewer. The family is likely to confer during the "break" and to return with their own work of addressing the future accomplished. Together, interviewers and family agree on the short-term psychotherapeutic approach to the case.

Rarely can we achieve an intervention in fewer than four interviews. In assisting the family with the presenting issues, our therapeutic goal is not only to relieve the symptom but also to address the family tensions and imbalance which the symptom represents. Our thesis is that even with a short-term therapeutic intervention, families can use their own strengths to face and master stress and developmental issues.

The C's were a rather sedentary couple. Dr. C, 40, was a medical researcher, while Mrs. C, 38, was a successful computer programmer who had been married eleven years before "she" could decide whether to have a baby. Now, she said, the baby was so all absorbing that she couldn't go back to work. Dr. C, whose role in the decision to have a child seemed to have been secondary, said that his research had stopped. Both parents were exhausted. Mrs. C complained that she could not sleep at night, couldn't let her baby cry, and couldn't leave Suzanna even in the daytime.

Suzanna was a pretty, curly-headed, and competent little girl. She pulled on furniture to stand up, looked for "lost objects" during the developmental exam, and elicited smiles from me. Actively exploring, she rarely looked back at her parents, although they called to her from time to time seeking a response. Suzanna gaily reached out to me, climbing on my leg to take my attention from her parents. What came across immediately was her competency, her sureness of herself with a stranger, and her almost constant searching, accompanied by delightful chortles. She gave the impression of a happy, cared-for, charming baby who expected to be responded to by those around her. Strikingly, she had little need to look back at her parents; she seemed to know, without any of the usual signaling, that her parents were there.

Dr. and Mrs. C, on the other hand, watched their daughter almost constantly—each parent shifting his or her body to face Suzanna as she cruised from one piece of furniture to another. I felt they showed remarkable restraint in not jumping to catch her when she teetered next to a piece of furniture. It was as if they *expected* her to manage for herself. They admired her achievements when I pointed them out, but took little credit for them, I felt. They talked about and looked at her as if she were some sort of unexpected miracle, for whom they'd done surprisingly little. They smiled at her achievements, but they did not hover over her, reprimand her, or seem self-conscious about her in any way.

During our interviews, Suzanna's parents kept watching her with obvious awe and pride. As soon as I commented on how great she was, they concurred. Mrs. C then added, "She's making our lives hell!" She said this with a smile which almost belied her words.

At this point, faced with the discrepancy between this glorious child's development and the parents' urgent request for help, I wondered what lay behind it all. Surely the only difficulty the child might present was her constant activity, her competence ("as if she didn't really need them"), her interest in everyone but her parents. She was not a truly hyperactive or destructive baby, but rather one who was "under a head of steam." Her behavior was so charming that one was sure she was not unloved.

Mrs. C's next statement seemed almost an answer to my associations. "I gave up so much to have her—and I wanted her to be perfect," she said. She quickly told me how successful she had been as a highly paid executive. Pointing to her husband she noted that her salary had been "equivalent to what he makes." Mrs. C told me what a struggle it had been even to consider "giving up her career" to have a baby; she had planned to be back at work three months after delivery.

But she hadn't been able to leave Suzanna. Mrs. C said:

> When I can't go back to work, I'm getting like my mother. I never wanted to be like her. She was a true hausfrau. I remember a time when I was 5 and my brother 2½, we were all going on a trip to the park. My mother got dressed up to come with us. My little brother said, "You belong in the kitchen. Stay at home. Father will take us." I realized then that women were supposed to be in the kitchen, and I never wanted to be like that. I got myself a Ph.D., married a researcher, and thought I was safe. Then I decided to have a baby. (She looked disapprovingly at her husband, who nodded rather passively.) When I knew I was really pregnant, I felt like I could do anything. I felt as if I was equal to conquering the world. That's why Suzanna's sleep problem is such a terrible blow. It's the first chink in my armor.

I picked up on this: "This makes you feel like you've failed?" She blushed, shifted uneasily, and looked at Suzanna. Her husband responded, "We've both failed." I said, "It must be a real problem for all of you." They replied, almost in chorus, "You just haven't any idea! That's why we are here. She *looks* so perfect. Only *we* know what she's really like."

Meanwhile, Suzanna had been showing me her rather precocious abilities. At 7 months, she stood and cruised around furniture with real competence. She took one hand off the furniture as if to show off. She gurgled and vocalized, "Hi" and "Dada" and "Ya!" in rapid succession. When we didn't get involved with her, she sat down to play with blocks. She was able to put one on top of the other. She took each toy, examined it (almost without looking at us), and used it correctly. I found myself in awe of her capacity to perform. She was not only competent but conscious of her skills; she seemed already to sense that she had an audience for her precocity. Yet there was nothing unattractive or eerie about her competence. I commented on the engaging quality of her behavior as well as on her ability to perform at a level several months beyond her age.

Dr. and Mrs. C responded, "You must see *us* as the problem. She's obviously so great that only we can ruin her." I said, "At least you must feel this. She almost seems to be showing me how great she is, and as if she doesn't need you." They took short breaths and looked at each other. Mrs. C said, "You've noticed it, too. From the first, I've been trying to insert myself, but she is so much a 'person.' She makes me feel as if I'm not even needed. It reminds me of how my brother made me feel when we were little." I said, "It seems to be almost a problem for you that Suzanna is so competent." "Well, I was, *too*, until she came along." At that point, Dr. C seemed to need to speak. He said, "She's really an amazing kid. But if she's so amazing, why are we having problems?" I looked at him quizzically, and he said, "It's us, isn't it?" I reminded them both that they'd each said something like that. I wondered if Suzanna made her parents feel helpless and not adequate to her.

Mrs. C said, "I never intended to be like my mother. She smothered us—me and my younger brother—with too much love. I always felt stifled by her. She couldn't let us go, and here I am doing the same thing with Suzanna." I wondered how she meant that. She said, "Oh, I watch her all day, and I go to her all night. She hasn't any chance to be herself."

Since I had been wondering whether such a pattern was at the root of Suzanna's sleep problem, I felt as if Mrs. C had suddenly read my mind. She said, "I know you are thinking that. I've read all your books. 'A sleep problem is the problem of the mother or father.' Well, it's *ours*. If I don't go to her, he will. So I have to beat him to it. And all the time we are both being dragged out. I can't go back to work. He can't do his research. We are both at the mercy of this baby." Mrs. C said all this with real vehemence. Meanwhile, Suzanna looked beatific as she played. Her father said, "What are we to do? We came to you because we knew you knew the answers. We've heard of your clinic and how they cure people's children."

At this point, I was tempted to give them the "solutions" they were looking for, but I believed the C's needed to be enabled to develop their own solutions, which I could then support or help them modify. Consequently, I turned the question back to the parents: "You must have had advice from many others." They told me of four or five people whom they had already consulted. One had told them to let Suzanna "cry it out"; one to sleep with her; another had suggested a medication, a fourth had let them know it was "all their fault," which they knew anyway. I commented that they already had many different kinds of advice and wondered why they thought none of it had worked. "You can see it's not her fault. Just look at her. We are the ones who are ruining her!"

I commented that the problem certainly didn't come from a lack of caring about Suzanna. They nodded vigorously. "What then is in your minds?" "Maybe we're not the right parents for her." "Tell me what you mean by that." "She needs younger, more flexible parents than we are." I commented that they seemed to feel their age was a real barrier. Mrs. C said, "We wanted this so much. We really wanted it to be perfect. She's perfect, but we're not." I said, "You seem to be always beating yourselves up for any failure in her. Not sleeping through isn't the worst failure a child can demonstrate." They nodded but said, "But more will follow." I said, 'It's almost as if you equate any failure as evidence that neither of you was adequate to do this job."

At this point Suzanna came up to my knee, stood up, and looked me in the face. It was impossible not to respond to her. As I did, both parents squirmed and Mrs. C's voice became almost childlike as she said, "You must tell me how to be a mother to this little monster." Dr. and Mrs. C both nodded vehemently. Since Mrs. C's immature-sounding voice and appeal seemed so out of context for these two very sophisticated people, I marked it in my mind as a critical point in our interview.

I said, "I don't know that I can tell you how to mother Suzanna. First of all, I'm very impressed at the kind of job you've done on your own. Whatever you may think, you are doing awfully well by her. But I think that isn't enough. You seem to feel the need to be perfect as parents for her. Any 'chink' is too much for you."

At this point, Mrs. C began almost to weep. She said, "I did so well before I tried this. I was competent. I loved my job. I felt as if I was a person. Now I'm not—all over again."

I asked her whether she wanted to comment on that. She said that she had known it would be hard, starting a family so late, but why should she care so much that she made herself fail. They had done everything right, planned everything carefully. They had a house and enough money. She had a job, and he had a brilliant career. They had gone to childbirth education classes, had "learned it all." She had a perfect pregnancy, but at the end, all their planning had failed and Suzanna had been born by caesarean section. She'd failed them from the first. "We haven't been equal to her," Mrs. C repeated, as if this were a chorus.

As Mrs. C talked, her voice shook with emotion. I commented on how deeply she cared about Suzanna and doing right by her. She assured me that she thought about her night and day.

She said her feelings toward Suzanna reminded her of her early relationship with her own mother, one which she had sworn never to reproduce. Everyone, said Mrs. C, criticized her mother for being a "typical Jewish mother." Now she understood the phenomenon all too well and was doing the same thing—"smothering Suzanna."

I wondered what she meant by smothering her. She said her own mother had made her feel helpless and inadequate. Mrs. C felt that she had either to be a female in the kitchen or to do something entirely different, to get away from her mother's model. "And now you are straddling the two models, and you feel you are failing," I said. The mother looked hard at me. At that point, as if she knew how involved her mother was getting, Suzanna fell and hit her hand slightly. She began to cry loudly. Mrs. C rushed to pick her up.

She tried rocking her in her arms, but Suzanna continued to scream. Mrs. C looked helplessly over the child's head and said, "Nighttime is like this. She screams as if with nightmares, then rocks herself in bed. I tried to let her cry like my pediatrician told me, but I just couldn't stand it. Her crying makes me weak and feel faint. Even if I could let her cry, her father couldn't." She looked for confirmation at Dr. C, who nodded. Then he said, "I can't stand it though. I can't get any work done either. Can we take a vacation—from her, I mean? We could leave her with Mrs. C's mother."

Meanwhile, I'd taken Suzanna to calm her down. She quieted immediately in my arms, started playing with my face and my clothing. She looked back at her mother reproachfully as if to say, "See, he knows how to quiet me."

Mrs. C looked at Suzanna, then at me, as if she felt very competitive and that I knew the baby better than she did. I sensed a real sadness in Mrs. C's look. I handed Suzanna back to her and said, "I think she needs you. She only came to me because she felt you weren't paying full attention to her. And now she's splitting us apart. So she's happy." Mrs. C looked at me with surprise. "You attribute real motives to her. She's only a baby." "Maybe you don't want to think of her as having thoughts of her own," I said, "You tell me you feel as if you are smothering her."

With that, Mrs. C put the baby down and said, "Suzanna, you can walk on your own." Suzanna accepted being put down, scurried over to my chair and pulled up to a standing position. Her mother watched her longingly.

All of this time, Dr. C had been almost completely silent. Now, as if given permission, he began to talk, not about how remarkable the baby was, but how much she'd disrupted their family. He spoke of the old adjustment before she came with real longing. "Now," he said, "she dominates our family."

When I tried to find out how much Dr. C had to do directly with Suzanna, Mrs. C almost immediately tried to take over the interview. I had to rephrase my question to Dr. C. He admitted that everything he tried to do, his wife could do better. I wondered whether he felt a bit unnecessary. He replied, "Except at night. Then my wife is so tired that I know she and the baby need me."

As Dr. and Mrs. C again spoke about Suzanna's apparently "perfect" development, I commented, "When she's less than ideal for you when you're alone, it must make you feel pretty guilty that you can be so angry with her and with each other." Mrs. C said, "The contrast lets us know where the problem is. But what can be done about it?" I responded that they would first have to let up on themselves and acknowledge that pitfalls and less-than-perfection were in the nature of parenting. I was sure that it was very hard to feel less than successful, but pointed out that any failure in Suzanna did not necessarily represent a failure in their parenting. In fact, although this might be hard for them to see or to allow, a "failure" might represent a sign of Suzanna as a separate individual.

I wondered whether Suzanna's nighttime waking wasn't recalling old conflicts for the C's about being independent, conflicts which they had dealt with earlier in their lives. I reminded them that having a baby presses one back into one's own past experience.

Mrs. C volunteered immediately, "Like being a woman means you're never your own, that you devote yourself to everyone around you, selflessly and tirelessly." I reminded her that had been her image of her mother, and one she'd had a hard time identifying with, but I wondered whether it needed to be an either/or situation. Mrs. C said, "It seems as if it must be. I guess I am afraid that any failure will threaten this wonderful situation we have." As she looked at her husband she added, "I've never been so much in love before, not even with you." He nodded imperceptibly as if he knew this already. Mrs. C continued, "Also, I feel a compulsion to be a good mother for her"—and with sudden insight—"as if any failure meant I might lose her." I confirmed this: "Or as if any failure meant you'd better split from her. Even by going back to work." She nodded her head vigorously, and her eyes filled with tears. I commented that separation seemed to be a pretty tortured problem for her.

Dr. C leaned forward to say, "I think that before Suzanna came, I was happy to have my wife be a successful professional. Now I want her at home with Suzanna, and, to be honest, I find I need more from her than I did before. I think I make her resent her role because I'm constantly asking for more from her, and at the same time, I'm competing with her for Suzanna. It's a funny and uncomfortable set of new roles. We weren't ready for all of this." "And when Suzanna doesn't make it easy at night it must really hit you between the eyes." "Yes!" they both chorused. "Each of you has fallen in love unexpectedly, and it's hard to let Suzanna become independent without feeling that you will be losing her completely. I think we'll need to work with each of you individually on some of the loss which this baby's independence means to you. As she gets more and more independent, it will be even harder for you." Mrs. C said, "What will we ever do when she's an adolescent and we're in our fifties?"

Although I knew they weren't worried about Suzanna's development, I suggested to the C's that I wanted to do a physical exam on her. In the course of the physical, I can usually tell a certain amount about social reaction, stranger anxiety, how both baby and parents handle stress. As a pediatrician, I find the physical exam is a paradigm so familiar that I can assess the child and parent's reactions all the time I am examining the child. Any individual difference in either child's or parent's behavior sets off a signal for me. During Suzanna's exam, her parents treated her as if she were much older, expecting her to sit on my table, to respond to my exam without any anxiety. She complied, and in fact was unusually cooperative, almost helping me to do my work. One got the feeling that this baby was already learning to nurture her parents. Yet there was little sign of this role costing her too much. I commented on this and wondered whether Suzanna's precocity during the day might be one reason she needed to break down at night. Her mother added, "It's so good to be needed by her that this makes it hard for us to leave her at night."

As we summed up the problem at the end of the session, it seemed to me that we were dealing with each of these parents' problems in separation from this charming, competent little girl. Not only was she unexpectedly winning, but she had struck at each of their feelings about their roles. She was so rewarding that neither of them wanted to share her, to leave her, or, in particular, to see her grow up. In unconscious ways, both parents were fostering her dependence at night. When we talked about separating or pushing Suzanna to be more independent by "learning" how to sleep through the night, each parent had real difficulties in contemplating a solution to the nighttime problem which involved giving up that much of her. In fact, when I summed up the work we needed to do to help them face the symptom which had brought them to the clinic, their reply was, "Could we go off on a two-week vacation and leave Suzanna with her grandparents?" I pointed out to them that they seemed to need to flee the problem or give up, rather than to face the problem and work on it themselves.

We planned three more sessions. One would be for mother, to work on her problems with separation and her competitive feelings about controlling and having this baby in an all-or-none situation. Another session would be for father, to help him with his own feelings about separation as well as with his role in supporting Mrs. C as she worked toward some separation from Suzanna. The third session would be used to sum up their experience with whatever regime was worked out in the earlier visits and then tested at home.

Second Session—With Mother

The second session was reserved for the mother. She came alone, immediately telling me how difficult it had been for her to leave Suzanna, who had sensed all morning that her mother was leaving her and had clung to her. When Mrs. C finally got ready to leave the house, Suzanna had completely fallen apart. She said this accusingly. I commented on Mrs. C's tone, saying: "I think you see me as a wedge that will separate you from Suzanna, even though you came to me because of your difficulties in allowing Suzanna to separate from you at night. Do you need for me to be the scapegoat? I think you are trying to tell me that you see separation as a major issue for you."

The mother smiled knowingly, as if I had indeed offered an insight to her. "I know. It's just so hard for me to lose any control over her. Losing her seems so final. If I can't control her, I may lose her completely. I waited so long before I dared to have her. I have such high expectations for her. Like myself. Except I want her to be perfect. I can't conceive of making mistakes with her." Mrs. C's emphasis on perfection seemed so unrealistic that I needed to comment again that parenting was not made up only of successes. Trying out approaches and experiencing and learning from failure were critical aspects of parenting.

At this point, Mrs. C's face clouded. She said, "But I don't *want* to be like my mother—always being soft and ineffectual." I asked whether she felt she had a difficult time with her own image as a woman like her mother. She repeated what she'd told me originally, that she'd always wanted to be different from her own mother, whom she saw as "the soft, feminine type, always giving to others, never protecting herself from pain or mistakes. Look at me. Here I am caught between trying not to be like her and being a perfectionist like myself."

I asked her how she thought she had become "a perfectionist." She said that she always thought her father was the one with high standards in the family. He was the disciplinarian and wanted "the world for his children." Her mother was more the dishevelled, dumpy housewife who tried strategies "to get us to sleep or to eat" but always seemed to be failing. "But," I said, "what was so painful about your mother's mothering?" She said, "Well, she ultimately lost. We became our own people, not hers." I wondered why Mrs. C associated this with "losing." She said, "Look at me. I didn't even want to be a woman like her." I said I wasn't so sure, but I did think that mothering came to her with some difficulty. She looked at me out of the corner of her eye: "Are you accusing me of being more maternal than I think I am?" I said, "I'm only going on the fact that Suzanna is really a delightful, charming little girl, and she didn't get it all from other people. Anyway, you've already told me how deeply you've fallen in love with her. Is that distinct from being maternal?"

She laughed appreciatively, and said, "Touché! I do love being a mother. But I'm so afraid of not being good at it." I wondered how much this fear had to do with being so sure of herself in another area and of having invested so much in being a perfectionist in her work. But I also thought that Mrs. C was struggling with deeper feelings about the pain involved in being a mother. She blushed, fell silent, then said, "I don't want to lose her. She's too precious to me." "Have you lost your own mother—or father—by becoming a person of your own?" "I guess I'd seen it as a sort of loss—when I was so invested in my work. When I go home, I have very little to say to my mother, but my father understands me exactly." I said, "Maybe you could let yourself get closer to your mother now and see what she went through in losing you, so she could help you let Suzanna go. For, as you've guessed, I see your sleep issues as being intimately tied up with Suzanna's autonomy. It's very tough for you to 'let' her learn about her own ability to comfort herself and learn to get down to sleep at night. However, as we talk, it's not only the sleep area but all areas of independence that are troublesome. It seems no coincidence to me that you come in for help when she is taking a real spurt in independence."

Her face softened as she said, "You make it sound so easy to see all of this. Why couldn't I have seen it for myself? I don't even feel it as bad. Somewhere I dreaded for you to be of any help, because I was so afraid it would be too painful if you found me a solution. Is this really a solution?"

I said that I wasn't at all sure that it was, for I hardly knew her, but I could see certain things in what she told me and in Suzanna that made it easy to recognize patterns that a lot of working women her age were struggling with. I thought she'd have to see whether they fit her or not. She said, "You mean I'm not unique? In a way I'm relieved. In another, I'm disappointed that my struggle isn't unique. It seemed so intense." I warned her that we had not solved her conflict. She would have to do the real work of sorting it out and seeing whether these were only a first layer of interpretations.

She said, "At least now I can leave my husband alone. I've been so angry with him that he couldn't help me or Suzanna. And when he was good with her, it made me even angrier. What's that all about?"

I said that I had sensed a certain amount of competition between them, and had wondered whether she understood it. "But," I said, "competition for a baby you care about is the nature of the game. However, maybe you wanted more from him than he could give—to either you or Suzanna." She said, "I felt it in terms of Suzanna. But maybe it was me. I really wanted him to pull me out of this tangle, and yet I knew he couldn't. I think ever since she came I felt he should fill a new role—not one I could really describe, but just a new one. He couldn't understand my faltering. He wanted to be more helpful and did step in and do all he could. He's been a wonderful father, but maybe that's the problem. He was too good at times, and when he was, I was jealous. I wanted him to see my side of it, not hers. When he was not good with Suzanna I felt, why can't he be someone else? Who's that someone else? I hate this competition—it takes me back to how I tried to cope with my feelings about my brother."

I commented that Mrs. C seemed to have an amazing amount of insight but that Suzanna's coming had really mobilized a lot of old conflicts for her. Some of them seemed painful and had been tough for her to face. But, in general, she seemed to have been using her own past experiences to give Suzanna a pretty good time. She said, "You've no idea what it means to me to hear that. I felt like a failure." She ended the interview for us by saying, "Well, you've certainly given me plenty to think about and to work on." I asked, "Did you want specific advice about handling the nighttime?" She replied, "I think I can find ways to do it. You've helped me see why I couldn't hear them or make them work."

I said, "Let me make two specific suggestions that might make your job easier. One, *do* teach Suzanna how to find a 'lovey' or a comforter to fall back on by herself. She's so competent, but it costs her a lot to be so independent. During the day, you can help her by pushing a teddy bear as a companion to fall back on when she's tired or frustrated. Then she'll have him with her at night, too. She might even be relieved to have her own way of getting herself back to sleep. The second is to wake her in the evening before she wakes you. Before you go to bed, rouse her, love her, and feed her; give her the lovey to cuddle. For some reason, if she feels comforted before she needs it, this makes a difference in the pattern. Anyway, when you do go back to work, you'll have this period to look forward to between you in the middle of the night."

Mrs. C seemed both more peaceful and energized than I'd seen her in our two sessions as she left.

Third Session—With Father

Dr. C came in jauntily asking "What did you do for my wife? She's been a different person since you saw her. She came home as if she'd conquered the world. All she could tell me was that she 'understood' herself. What kind of miracle is that? Can you do it for me? She's been so sure of herself that I can hardly recognize her. She puts Suzanna to bed at night; they both hug each other and are even glad to see each other go. Suzanna has been sleeping through almost every night since she was here. That is, she sleeps after my wife wakes her. They seem to have such a nice time now. I'm rather jealous."

I wondered what he felt jealous about. He said, "At first, it was of you for helping her when I couldn't. Now, I think it's that she and Suzanna are having such an easy time. Before, it was me and Suzanna. Now it's her mother. I think I want Suzanna to like me best, and this new, easy role is making Suzanna seem so happy with her mother." I commented that it sounded as if he'd almost gotten a bit of vicarious pleasure out of Mrs. C's failure. He protested, but he said, "At least it gave me a role. If they're too comfortable, they might not need me." I assured him that would never be so. I'd seen how Suzanna needed and relied on him, and I knew from what she'd told me, how much his wife needed him. I wondered whether it wasn't just painful shifting roles.

"Well, it is for me. I never had much of a father, or even much of a childhood. My father was away working all the time. I was an only child, so I had to fill all my mother's needs. She wanted me to be perfect. I had to do everything she wanted or she threatened me with falling apart. I always felt as if I were her only reason for living. That's a helluva way to grow up. It made me a perfectionist. It also made me a lonely, lonely person. Before I met my wife, I'd never had a close relationship with anyone." "Except your mother?" "That was too close. That wasn't even a relationship. I was just overpowered. I can remember her feeding me when I was 3 or 4. She made me eat. She even slept in my room until I was 8 or so. I never had a childhood."

I wondered how he'd been able to free himself up as much as he did. I reminded him of my observation with Suzanna—that he'd been able to let her explore, find her way around the room without hovering. And, in a way, he'd given her a good deal of freedom.

"But not when she cries, or at night. And, in fact, any time she shows any slight need for me, I feel gratified. I want to hover over her, but she won't let me. She's too strong."

I commented that he seemed to be surrounded by strong women. He laughed and said, "I need them more than they need me. I guess I feel completely in love with Suzanna. Suddenly she seems the answer to all my dreams. I'd never had such a miraculous relationship before. Now I know I've got to let her go. What can I replace her with?"

I thought his wife certainly needed him, for she was having trouble giving Suzanna her autonomy too. Dr. C said, "But she seems to enjoy her even more now that she's come to peace with her."

"And you don't feel it, do you?" "Well, I feel jealous. I want them to need me—not each other. And, yet, I've been the one who wanted my wife to stay at home with her. As long as she's there, I feel as if Suzanna is safe. If she goes back to work, who knows? We might lose her."

I asked him to talk about this feeling of potential loss, the sense that if Suzanna were not totally dependent on her parents she would be totally lost to them. Dr. C replied, "I just feel so empty when I'm away from her. I'm afraid she won't be there for me." "Have there been any big losses for you before?" "Not real ones. I always dreamed—or wished—that I'd had a brother or sister. And I felt as if I'd lost him or her when I was growing up. I felt as if I'd done something bad, and I deserved to be my mother's only child. I guess I really hated that role more than I was aware of."

I pointed out how hard it had been for him to deal with his own struggle for autonomy. No wonder Suzanna's was hard for him. I saw his involvement with her as a natural result of having "fallen in love with her." I reminded him that both he and Mrs. C had told me that on the first visit and that this experience seemed to have come as a surprise, or even as a miraculous revelation.

He grinned at me and said, "Surely it's not that simple!" I assured him it wasn't at all, but that a baby did touch off the deep struggles in all of us, and that he'd obviously done awfully well for Suzanna. Now it was time to work to get onto a new stage with her. I repeated what I'd said to Mrs. C, that Suzanna's burgeoning independence was delightful but so difficult for them, each for his or her own reason, that I thought that was why they'd come at this time.

He said, "You know, I think we've lived on the miraculous part of having her at our advanced ages, and now we're having to adjust to the other side of it—that having a baby means being able to give her up in stages. I do feel as if I can do it. I'm not sure why. I guess I just want to do it right. I care too much about her. Now you've helped me see that I can do best by her if I support my wife when she needs it and give Suzanna her head to grow up. I've never really felt so useful or 'so much like a person.' I'm proud to feel like a father."

Fourth Visit

When Suzanna was 11 months old the whole C family came to the clinic. Suzanna came dancing in, looking well put together. She looked back at her parents for approval, took toys to them for help, and allowed them to join in her achievements.

Mrs. C began: "I have been able to see her side of it at last—like you wanted me to. I realize that I was too caught up with my own problems—working, my own struggles with femininity, letting her go. Your letting me cry on your shoulder let me see that I can be a baby and a mother at the same time. Our marriage is different. We have begun to be able to talk to each other; I can ask him to help me. He even loves it."

Dr. C added, "I feel like a person who can help my girls. She has let me tell her what to do. She lets me put Suzanna to bed now. On bad nights, I take over and comfort Suzanna first, then tell her now it's time to go to sleep by yourself. She does! I feel like a beast, but I also feel like I'm in charge. It's a feeling I haven't had before except when I got through medical school or when I published a paper. Amazing! Now it's with people, and I feel powerful. I no longer need to wonder at my feelings of competitiveness with my wife. We've begun to sort ourselves out. Suzanna is sleeping, eating, and we're loving her independence. It's like a miracle, and we feel like a family. Thank you."

I wondered whether it hadn't been almost too easy to help them. I wondered what might happen the next time they hit a snag with her. They looked at each other, and Mrs. C said, "I think we feel on a different level of competence. We really faced this, and you helped us work it out. But we really feel *we* worked it out—as a family. Can't we do the same thing next time?"

I assured them that I could help if they needed me but that I really felt as if they had dealt with their problems *with* Suzanna and *for* her, and I felt that was pretty great. Suzanna certainly seemed to show it, as, aglow, she cruised around the room.

Discussion

Complex interactions among many factors influence the development of parent–infant relationships. A young baby has the power to stir up traces of a variety of early childhood experiences; these memories shape not only the parents' plans for how they will care for their infant but also the unconsciously motivated behaviors that contribute to each parent's individual caregiving style. Another powerful factor influencing parent–infant relationships is the infant's individual temperament or behavioral style. The impact of differences among infants has been studied extensively and is accepted as common knowledge by an increasing percentage of middle-class American families.

These psychological determinants of parent–infant relationships are widely illustrated in the transactions between Suzanna and her parents. Indeed, were it not for the description of the physical examination of Suzanna, one could imagine the interviews with Dr. and Mrs. C taking place in any number of profesional settings, conducted by a psychologist, a social worker, or another mental health professional. In fact one might wonder whether pediatricians should be in the business of offering interpretive statements of the kind recorded here to parents.

It is important to remember that the intervention with Dr. and Mrs. C and Suzanna took place in a clinical setting where intervention is kept brief by plan and pitched at a pragmatic level, even though it is based on the staff's knowledge of the complex, dynamic events that characterize human relationships. This knowledge base, combined with a range and depth of clinical experience, suggests to the pediatrician when it is appropriate to go beyond the usual pediatric contact in discussing a normal developmental crisis with a family. In this case, the fact that psychological issues were both close to the surface of the couple's awareness and attached to appropriate affect indicated to the clinician that a light touch would be effective. Had Suzanna or her parents looked different at the follow-up visit, a referral for longer-term treatment might have been made.

We must remember, too, that their psychological self-awareness notwithstanding, Dr. and Mrs. C chose to come with their concerns about Suzanna not to a mental health practitioner but to a pediatric clinic. "We've heard of your clinic," Dr. C said on the first visit, "and how they cure people's children." Even the experienced pediatrician was tempted, faced with this plea/demand/challenge, to offer a "solution" or "cure" for Suzanna's sleep disturbance. The decision to work instead toward helping the couple find their own solutions to a developmental issue through a process designed to foster their feelings of competence as parents reflects a changing view of the pediatrician's role.

It is worth examining changing expectations of the pediatrician in the context of the social environment of infant care in the United States today.

A New Definition of "Survival" in Infancy

For the American middle class, the concept of survival in infancy has been redefined. Physical health is assumed. The timely achievement of developmental milestones is expected. The "new viability" demands a guarantee that the young child develops abilities that will assure success in a highly competitive world of limited resources and fairly unpredictable change. While our ancestors worried about adequate nutrition, contemporary parents worry about whether their babies are receiving sufficient mental nurturance to facilitate their intellectual development. Energies that used to focus on sterilizing bottles and preparing the right formula are now expended on selecting the most educationally beneficial mobile for a newborn. Curricula originally designed to promote skill acquisition in developmentally vulnerable or disabled infants are now adapted to accelerate the development of competence in all babies. Data demonstrating the relative plasticity of the immature central nervous system provide fuel for those who advocate structured "early intervention" for everyone. For increasing numbers of American parents, raising a healthy child with normal development is not enough. Their goal is nothing less than precocity and competitive advantage. Whereas pediatricians of the nineteenth and early twentieth centuries cautioned against too much stimulation in the early months, many contemporary parents apply pressure regarding performance from birth on.

Middle-class professional adults who, like Suzanna's parents, carefully plan their first pregnancy and parenthood as they reach the middle adult years may be particularly vulnerable to such new concepts of infant "survival."

The postponement of parenthood is itself a reflection of both advanced technology and social change. Effective contraception, the option of therapeutic abortion, and evolving techniques of in-vitro fertilization have created an unprecedented opportunity for personal influence over the timing of childbearing. What was once inevitable and variably planned has been transformed into a carefully calculated life option. While clinical medical achievements have made delayed childbearing possible, social change has made it preferable for many. For women, whose aspirations beyond motherhood are increasingly supported, the issue of work outside the home has become broadened to embrace the concept of full career development. For men, whose investment in parenting responsibilities increasingly extends beyond the role of provider to that of nurturer, the balance between career and family needs demands careful planning and negotiation. For both men and women, changing expectations of what life can offer, and interaction among agendas of personal identity, intimacy, and career, all demand time for resolution before one is ready to assume the responsibility of parenthood.

The Burden of Competency

New parenthood, whenever it occurs, is a humbling experience. The immediate need to master an incredible array of seemingly mundane tasks, coupled with the simultaneous negotiation of personal psychological realignments, presents a major life challenge. Successful adults are particularly vulnerable as they confront the realities of infant care. Suzanna's mother, for example, was a "highly paid executive" whose initial reaction to learning of her pregnancy was a feeling that, "I could do anything . . . as if I was equal to conquering the world." She had forgotten what inexperience felt like; failure was an unfamiliar feeling. The intrapsychic issues that the experience of motherhood stirred up had remained relatively well managed in her previous adult roles as a computer programmer and spouse. In some respects, it is ironic that her years of success as an achieving adult made her more vulnerable and less well prepared for the struggle of parenthood. When told that she seemed to be having a problem with Suzanna's competence, her mother said, "Well, I was [competent] *too*, until she came along."

The issue of competence, although salient for both parents, has different implications for contemporary men and women. For men, whose own fathers often played peripheral roles in their early childhood, the struggle often revolves more around their degree of participation in child rearing rather than their level of competence. Consequently they can gain self-esteem simply from their willingness to "try" and to "help out." In the minds of mothers, however, there is no acceptable substitute for mastery. At a time when career-oriented success has become so important, many women find the traditional tasks of mothering more difficult to master than the professional demands of their work outside the home. Indeed, even if the chores of modern parenthood may be shared equally, the psychological burden of assuring competent childrearing remains with the mother, whose access to resources and support may be more tenuous than ever before.

The Myth of Perfectability

The wish for a perfect infant and the pressure to be a perfect parent are closely related to the burden of competence. When confronted with her need to be a perfect parent, Suzanna's mother cried: "I did so well before I tried this. I was competent. I loved my job. I felt as if I was a person. Now I'm not—all over again." In touching upon issues with her own mother, Mrs. C highlights the current equation of competence with perfection. In a society where the decision to not have children is increasingly acceptable, and where the carefully planned baby is unlikely to have many siblings, each infant represents an enormous narcissistic investment for his or her parents. Suzanna's mother admits: "I waited so long before I dared to have her. I have such high expectations for her. Like myself. Except I want her to be perfect. I can't conceive of making mistakes with her." When Suzanna's parents insist, "You can see it's not her fault. Just look at her. We are the ones who are ruining her," one wonders whether they need to see the problem in themselves because that is less threatening than the thought that their daughter might not be "perfect."

One has a sense that Dr. and Mrs. C may have sought out someone whom they saw as the "perfect pediatrician" to help them reestablish "paradise." It was the task of the pediatrician in this case, as it is the challenge facing other clinicians who work with infants and families, to use his knowledge, experience, sensitivity, and skills to promote adaptive—not perfect—family relationships.

Lessons and Challenges

Child-rearing attitudes and practices are influenced by an array of intrapsychic and cultural forces. Attitudes toward infants and their care change with the changing values of the society. Growing contemporary trends emphasize cognitive stimulation, early competitive advantage, and an anxious striving for perfection in the face of an unpredictable and somewhat threatening future.

Socialization of young children during a period of rapid change is difficult. When fundamental adult roles are complicated by social revolution, the task can be overwhelming. For previous generations of mothers, a need for defining new roles and seeking alternative commitments came in their late thirties and forties when the nest was empty. Many women today establish a well-defined professional identity in what used to be thought of as the childbearing years; for them motherhood is a midlife challenge. For fathers, who continue to assume the major responsibilities of economic support, intimacy with their children and nurturing competence have become less of a hobby and more of a personal imperative. Shifting concepts of femininity, masculinity, motherhood, and fatherhood, and the scarcity of role models impose a weighty burden.

The task of the clinician is to identify and understand interactions among the multiple determinants of individual behavior in families with young children. The pediatrician is particularly well situated to promote adaptive family relationships through the anticipatory guidance that forms the cornerstone of contemporary child health care.

6

A Stitch in Time: Using Emotional Support, Developmental Guidance, and Infant–Parent Psychotherapy in a Brief Preventive Intervention

Jeree H. Pawl, Ph.D.

The case of Bonita and her parents highlights the value of prompt intervention when difficulties in the interaction between child and parents already exist and relationships in the entire family seem likely to deteriorate and become further distorted. In this instance a further order of preventive work was also possible, because the family included a newborn infant who could directly benefit from the intervention focused on the parents and older child. The methods of intervention were those developed by Selma Fraiberg and her colleagues in Michigan (Fraiberg, 1980) and further elaborated at the Infant–Parent Program of the University of California, San Francisco (Lieberman, 1983; Pawl and Pekarsky, 1983; Lieberman and Pawl, 1984). These methods center on flexible intervention services which are typically home-based and include the parent(s) and infant together. Home visiting offers the most efficient and richest context for the observation and understanding of the functioning of a child and family. Only through home visits can one fully appreciate the shape and texture of a family's daily existence and their experience of one another.

Treatment consists of a flexible mix of concrete and emotional support, developmental guidance, and infant–parent psychotherapy. Concrete support, in the form of guiding families to services or actually providing service, such as transportation to appointments or to a location for food, is clearly helpful. This effort may also represent the only form of concern or help that a family can initially experience. Other families can accept from the beginning as emotionally supportive the therapist's understanding, interest, and investment in the family.

Throughout this process the infant or toddler remains the focus of the treatment. Information regarding the socioaffective development of a child is offered nondidactically in response to parental concerns as they emerge in the course of the work. Parents' conflicts with the child are seen in the light of the contribution made by their own past experiences to their current experience of the child. The degree to which these kinds of efforts are utilized in a particular intervention depends upon what is necessary and possible in the particular situation. In the following case, developmental guidance was the primary mode of intervention.

Case Presentation

Bonita and her parents, Mr. and Mrs. Lopez, were referred to the Infant–Parent Program when Bonita was 2 years, 5 months of age. A sibling had just been born. The family was referred by Dr. Forrest, the pediatrician who was following Bonita at a city-county hospital. Some months previously there had been medical concern about Bonita involving an obscure syndrome. A number of tests had been performed, though none was significantly intrusive. The syndrome was finally ruled out. However, Dr. Forrest was seriously concerned because Bonita showed severe behavior problems during clinic visits, and her mother had confirmed that Bonita was a serious problem at home. Mrs. Lopez indicated that she felt helpless to deal with her daughter's behavior.

Because of a language barrier, Dr. Forrest had few details of the family's background or current life, though she knew that Mrs. Lopez had emigrated from South America with her husband several years before. What the pediatrician could observe in the clinic, however, was extremely worrisome. Dr. Forrest described Bonita as having frequent tantrums. Often Bonita came in to the examining room and immediately hid in a corner. At other times she was extremely passive but then would alternately engage in wild screaming and desperate clinging to her mother. Occasionally, Bonita would stop screaming very abruptly without any perceptible intervention, and then, just as inexplicably, she would hurl herself against a wall, glare angrily at her mother, and thrash and scream. According to Dr. Forrest, Mrs. Lopez was clearly very embarrassed by Bonita's behavior, but appeared unable to respond.

Mrs. Lopez had reported to Dr. Forrest that at home Bonita had often awakened screaming at night and could not be consoled. Frequently, Mrs. Lopez or her husband would stay up all night trying to soothe their daughter, a process which exhausted them all. Mrs. Lopez said that Valium had been prescribed earlier by one pediatrician, but she was reluctant to try it and had not done so. Eventually, even without medication, Bonita's night terrors had begun to subside somewhat.

As this family spoke only Spanish, a bilingual and bicultural therapist from the Infant–Parent Program was assigned; through an interpreter, Dr. Forrest informed the mother that she could expect a call from someone from the Infant–Parent Program who might be useful in understanding Bonita's behavior.

Initial Home Visits: The Assessment Period

With every case referred, the Infant–Parent Program conducts an initial assessment, usually consisting of four or five home visits and one office visit over a period of about a month. The office visit includes a videotaped developmental assessment of the infant or toddler and a free play sequence between child and parents. The functioning of the family is understood to express the unique contributions of each member to the family's transactions. An effort is made to understand each family member's unique history and the context of his or her culture, subculture, and socioeconomic surround; these determine the nature of family transactions.

The assessment process is designed to evaluate not only the child's affective, social, and cognitive functioning and the quality of the parents' caregiving practices, but also, and more important, the parents' willingness to accept intervention and their ability to use it on behalf of the baby. In this sense, the assessment process has a built-in and very deliberate element of intervention. By carefully timed comments, including clarifications and interpretations, and by close monitoring of the parents' responses, we gather information about the potential use of emotional support, developmental guidance, or more introspective approaches for a family.

The initial visit with the Lopez family was a home visit, arranged by phone. During the phone call the mother reported that she was exhausted, worried about Bonita, and eager for help. On the day of the visit, Mrs. Lopez answered the door. A small child stood behind her, peering sullenly at the therapist. Mrs. Lopez was small, slender, and pretty, but she looked strained and exhausted. The therapist established that the child was indeed Bonita, introduced herself, and explained that she would be talking to her mommy but also would like to get to know her. Mrs. Lopez led the therapist directly to a bedroom. Bonita, a well-developed, pretty child with a wary, sullen expression, followed but kept her distance.

In the bedroom were two twin-sized beds and a crib in which 2-week-old Cecelia was sleeping. When Mrs. Lopez offered the therapist a peek at the baby, Bonita began running wildly from bedroom to living room to dining room and back. Mrs. Lopez told her to stop running and to sit down, but her instructions were without any effect. After the therapist and Mrs. Lopez seated themselves in the bedroom, Bonita continued to run from room to room and finally hurled a toy at the therapist. Mrs. Lopez screamed at Bonita that she couldn't do things like that and that she was to stop running, but she made no actual move to control her.

The therapist commented that she guessed that it was just this kind of thing that Mrs. Lopez was concerned about and that she, the therapist, was there to think with her about these difficulties. Mrs. Lopez agreed. The therapist then commented that just now the behavior seemed to have begun when she and Mrs. Lopez had admired Cecelia. Mrs. Lopez replied by launching into a lengthy description of how her pregnancy seemed to have changed Bonita. She said she had begun to have a very difficult time with her daughter then. As her condition had become more obvious, Bonita had often hit her very hard in the stomach and had become very angry and violent at any mention of the baby that was coming. From the midpoint of the pregnancy on, Bonita, who had been previously very attached to her mother, refused to allow Mrs. Lopez to have anything to do with her and developed a dramatic preference for her father. During the night, Bonita would awaken screaming, and toward the end of the pregnancy would reject her mother's comfort and could only be consoled by the father. Mrs. Lopez could offer no explanation for Bonita's rage at her mother's pregnancy, other than that the little girl was angry and jealous about the baby. The therapist commented on how difficult this all was, and Mrs. Lopez agreed that both she and her husband felt that Bonita was "impossible" and that "something was very wrong with her." The therapist's offer to meet with both Mrs. Lopez and her husband seemed worthwhile to Mrs. Lopez, but she said that as Mr. Lopez worked all day during the week she didn't know how this could happen. The therapist suggested that some Saturday might work, and Mrs. Lopez said that it certainly would.

Meanwhile, Bonita continued to burst into the room briefly, sometimes jumping on the bed, and once throwing a toy iron across the room the moment after her mother warned her not to. Mrs. Lopez was absolutely unable to control Bonita's behavior; occasionally she asked her to be quiet and sit down and later she begged her to do so, but these appeals were ineffective. Questioning revealed that although there were no toys anywhere in sight, there were some playthings in a box in a closet. Mrs. Lopez never got them out, and she seemed too exhausted to reflect on how Bonita could occupy herself acceptably.

Mrs. Lopez explained to the therapist that it was not their flat. They rented only the bedroom. The rest of the flat belonged to a family with four children ages 6 through 10. The woman, Mrs. Rodriguez, also cared for a 2-year-old boy whose mother worked. Mrs. Rodriguez and the little boy could occasionally be heard and seen in the rest of the flat. Bonita, according to Mrs. Lopez, interacted with this child and the other children primarily by fighting. Mrs. Lopez felt that though the 2-year-old day care child was four months younger than Bonita, he was much brighter and far better behaved than her daughter. Mrs. Lopez then explained that she and her family had lived with the Rodriguez family for the last two months after living by themselves for the two previous months. Before that, Mrs. Lopez and Bonita had stayed with her mother 400 miles away while Mr. Lopez had worked in this area. This had been necessary because it was the only place that Mr. Lopez had been able to find work, but the separation had been very difficult for Mrs. Lopez. During this conversation Bonita flopped down next to her mother and her mother caressed her briefly and awkwardly. The therapist engaged Bonita briefly from a distance and then Bonita left the room, picked up two dirty glasses from the sink and returned, offering one glass to the therapist. The therapist pretended to drink and thanked Bonita. Bonita smiled for the first time.

As Mrs. Lopez and the therapist made arrangements for the next week's visit, Mrs. Lopez mentioned some hospital appointments she had set up the next week for both Cecelia and Bonita. As the therapist stood up, Bonita began crying and clinging to her mother. The therapist bent down to Bonita and told her that she was leaving now, that she would see her at home again and not at the hospital, and that they would play a little if she liked. Bonita continued to cry and Mrs. Lopez made no attempt to console her. The therapist and Mrs. Lopez agreed to meet early in the morning so that the therapist could get a sense of the usual activities of the entire household.

At the next visit Mrs. Lopez answered the door with Bonita again behind her, silent and staring, with her diapers soaked and hanging to her knees. From the kitchen came the noise of the Rodriguez children hurrying to prepare for school. The day care boy was wandering aimlessly around the flat.

Bonita did not follow Mrs. Lopez and the therapist into the bedroom but stayed in the dining room and kitchen. At one point she brought a chessboard and pieces into the room and placed them near the therapist, then

quickly scurried out. Twice her mother yelled at her to
return the chess equipment as it belonged to the other
family. The therapist said that it must be very hard for
Bonita to be clear about what she could play with and what
she couldn't. Mrs. Lopez replied in a hopeless tone that
Bonita was very destructive with toys anyway and didn't
really like to play with them.

Throughout this visit, Bonita kept her distance despite her mother's encouragement to come into the bedroom. The therapist repeatedly assured both Mrs. Lopez
and Bonita that they should go about their business normally and that there would be time later for the therapist
to get to know Bonita. She said that Bonita did not have
to interact or play with the therapist until she wanted to.
Bonita did not play with the Rodriguez children or the 2-
year-old. She moved incessantly from one object to another, most of which were forbidden to her. She didn't
speak to anyone but expressed herself solely by crying or
screaming when her activities were disrupted.

The level of chaos in the house was notable. In response to a discussion about this, Mrs. Lopez said that she
would enjoy bringing Bonita to the playroom at the Infant-
Parent Program. She and the therapist agreed that after
one more home visit Mrs. Lopez would come with Bonita
to the office. Mrs. Lopez also said her husband would be
able and very willing to come to the office some Saturday.
Mrs. Lopez and the therapist agreed to discuss this during
the next visit.

At the third home visit, Bonita again stood near her
mother when Mrs. Lopez answered the door, and stared
sullenly at the therapist. Both Mrs. Lopez and Mrs. Rodriguez were eating breakfast at the kitchen table, and the
therapist was given a chair off to the side and offered some
juice. During the next fifteen minutes Bonita hovered in
the doorway, looking at the therapist, but she dashed away

at any responsive glance or remark. Her mother encouraged Bonita to join them. Again the therapist said there was no rush; when Bonita was ready they would get to know one another.

In answer to questions about Bonita's usual behavior with strangers, Mrs. Lopez explained with much concern that not only was Bonita extremely hesitant with unfamiliar people, but she did not seem to be able to get comfortable even with more familiar people. For example, if Bonita were left alone with Mrs. Rodriguez, she would scream, tremble, and cry desperately. Mrs. Lopez said she thought Bonita must not be as intelligent as other children who seemed able to manage such situations. The therapist replied that it must be very difficult for Mrs. Lopez to feel sympathetic to Bonita when the child made such demands on her. Mrs. Lopez softened somewhat and said that it had not always been that way; she could remember when Bonita played quite happily by herself and didn't always need her attention every minute.

In response to the therapist's question, Mrs. Lopez said that having found Bonita increasingly impossible during her pregnancy, she had finally reached the point of feeling completely helpless, ineffectual, and almost indifferent to her daughter. What she remembered of a good relationship was ruined. Mrs. Lopez seemed very sad and sighed hopelessly. Things were no smoother now that the baby was born; they were worse. Mrs. Lopez worried about Bonita hurting the baby. Bonita tried to climb into the crib and was heedless of the damage she might inflict. Occasionally she threw things at the baby.

Mrs. Rodriguez spoke up and said that it was very difficult for Mrs. Lopez to have a child who was so clinging and demanding of her attention. She agreed with Mrs. Lopez that Bonita must have a "bad temperament" and that this was the reason she did not "mind" her mother or play nicely with the other children in the household. Asked about her experiences with Bonita, Mrs. Rodriguez said that Bonita would not let her approach too closely and would scream or cry if she tried to pick the child up or put her on her lap. She reported that when Mrs. Lopez was seven months pregnant, Bonita had stayed the entire week with the Rodriguez family and it had been miserable for them all. Bonita would cry all day long until her father came home from work, and then she would cry again when he left to visit Mrs. Lopez in the hospital. The therapist responded that she had not known that Mrs. Lopez had been hospitalized. Mrs. Lopez sighed and said that she had been very ill and that it was an awful time. The therapist then wondered if this were especially difficult for Bonita, as well, and wondered if the toddler had understood where her mother was. Mrs. Lopez said Bonita came once or twice to the hospital, but it didn't seem to help. "Besides," she added, "Bonita screamed and cried when she came with me for my check-ups. She trembled and clung to me and started screaming when we got there. It started almost as soon as I found out I was pregnant."

As the adults talked, Bonita went in and out of the kitchen. If the therapist looked at her, she would whine and run away. Once Bonita approached a bit closer and stood with a book in her hand. The therapist asked if she could see the book. Bonita hesitated and then handed her the book—quickly running away. Mrs. Lopez tried to insist that she remain, but the therapist suggested that they just let Bonita be in charge.

At this point, another woman who was a regular visitor to the household arrived with her 2½-year-old boy, Roberto. Greetings were exchanged, and the therapist was introduced. The visitor made herself comfortable and joined the conversation. She too sympathized with Mrs. Lopez in having a child with such a "bad temperament," one who clung to her mother all the time when she tried to do her chores. The little boy hesitated only briefly before initiating interaction with the therapist. All of the women pointed out how friendly and verbal he was and how confident. Mrs. Lopez said wistfully that she wished Bonita were like that. The therapist sympathized with Mrs. Lopez' concern but pointed out that each individual has his or her own way. She said that it also seemed as if Bonita had had hard times with separation and that Mrs. Lopez' pregnancy might have meant to her primarily the occasion for more separations. The therapist added that nonetheless "it must be very hard to see someone like Roberto and then be patient with Bonita's difficulties." Mrs. Lopez replied, "I feel very angry sometimes and I worry that this is just the way she is, that something is really wrong with her." The therapist said they would see if they could work together to understand Bonita and try to make changes.

Following this conversation, Bonita entered the room and wanted to be picked up. Mrs. Lopez did so, and then stood rocking to and fro while Bonita buried her head in her mother's neck. Mrs. Lopez attempted to induce Bonita to talk to the therapist. The therapist responded by empathizing with Bonita, saying that it must be hard for her to have the therapist come and feel that everyone wanted Bonita to talk or play with her, and then to hear everyone talking about Bonita. It was confirmed that for the next meeting they would meet at the Infant–Parent Program's playroom so that the therapist, Bonita, and Mrs. Lopez could have a little more privacy. This remained very agreeable to Mrs. Lopez.

By this point in the assessment, it was clear to the therapist that the relationship between Mrs. Lopez and Bonita was a very troubled one. Bonita behaved in an angry way much of the time, and Mrs. Lopez was either angry in response or depressed and overwhelmed. The therapist felt that Mrs. Lopez' hospitalization during pregnancy and the prolonged loss of Mr. Lopez by both mother and child had played a significant role in the difficulties

now being experienced. What had been a positive relationship had been destroyed over the past several months, and
this needed to be further understood.

Program Visits: Treatment

As Bonita and Mrs. Lopez approached the waiting
room at the Infant–Parent Program, Bonita noticed the
shelf of toys, and her face lit up with interest. Almost
immediately, however, she saw the therapist, and her smile
faded. She stopped walking, assumed a sullen expression,
grabbed her mother, and began whining. Mrs. Lopez and
Bonita were invited by the therapist into the playroom.
Bonita began to cry as her mother deftly extricated herself
and walked in while Bonita stood outside, immobile but
crying. Her mother turned and began to pull and push
Bonita into the room. The therapist suggested that they
simply sit in view of Bonita and invite her in. Bonita was
told that she didn't have to come in but that she was truly
welcome and could play with the toys in the room. She
continued to cry. All were in sight of one another, and
after a few minutes Bonita ran swiftly to her mother,
where she continued crying. Mrs. Lopez assured Bonita
that the therapist wasn't going to do anything to her, but
she comforted her in no other way. Bonita hid her face in
her mother's lap and cried desperately. Mrs. Lopez
seemed utterly helpless and alternately encouraged and
scolded Bonita. The therapist said she thought that for
whatever reason Bonita seemed desperately unhappy and
frightened, and asked Mrs. Lopez if she thought perhaps
just some consolation from her mother would help her
some. Mrs. Lopez then offered her lap to Bonita and began to rock her and speak calmly to her. The crying lasted
for fifteen minutes.

During that time, Mrs. Lopez said that this was what
Bonita did when they went to the main hospital building

for any purpose. "Bonita begins crying as soon as she sees the doors." On questioning, Mrs. Lopez revealed that she had often lied to Bonita about whether the hospital trip was for her, her sister, her mother, or to pay a medical bill, because Bonita would calm somewhat if assured it was not for her directly. She added that Bonita would often cry this way at home if she suddenly realized that Mrs. Lopez was even in another room. Again the therapist underlined the issue of separation for Bonita and how fearful she seemed to be of so many things that might mean her mother would somehow be lost to her.

At the end of fifteen minutes, Bonita was briefly responsive to the therapist. Choosing from among all the toys, she brought the therapist a toy telephone. After peeking up under her brows to see what was happening, Bonita approached another toy phone at some distance from the therapist and said, "Hello." Suddenly she was overwhelmed again and fled back to her mother, clinging and sobbing hysterically. In answer to the therapist's questions as to what Bonita's experience with telephones had been, Mrs. Lopez said that during her pregnancy—from the fourth to seventh month—she and Bonita had lived away from the father. While he had remained here in the city working, they had stayed with Mrs. Lopez' mother. Mrs. Lopez reported that Bonita would sometimes talk to her father on the telephone but that she never saw him. She spoke at length about how much she had missed her husband and added that she had been quite lonely and depressed.

The therapist wondered if Bonita might also have been missing Mr. Lopez a lot. She asked whether the fact that her mother was so unhappy was something that Bonita had been sensitive to, as well. Mrs. Lopez said she supposed it was true, that she hadn't thought of it that way. She said that when they were together again, Bonita really preferred her father. This had not been true at all when Bonita was a baby or even before Mrs. Lopez became pregnant, but now Bonita definitely had a preference for her father. When he was around she went to him for everything. Asked how that made her feel, Mrs. Lopez said that it irritated her and seemed unfair, but also that she got so she really didn't care. What she cared about was that Bonita was so impossible and wild and wouldn't mind her.

From the safety of her mother's lap, Bonita again gradually began watching the therapist and finally stopped crying. When accompanied by her mother, she was able to approach some toys located at a distance from the therapist, but she howled if her mother tried to leave and sit in her chair again. Mrs. Lopez showed no inclination to play with Bonita as she used the toys, even when encouraged. She repeatedly attempted to leave Bonita, who would then begin crying. These interactions were described and highlighted in a neutral way by the therapist.

In response to a question, Mrs. Lopez said Bonita almost never really played with toys but would sometimes play near her in the kitchen with cookware. The therapist immediately got out the toy stove, dishes, and pans, and invited Bonita to help cook and set the table. Bonita gradually approached the therapist, though with great suspicion and tremendous caution. She was clumsy in her play, frequently whimpered, and finally, after ten minutes or so, began crying again and rushed to her mother. As the therapist started to pick up the toys, Bonita voluntarily passed a plate to her and then picked up a cup at the therapist's invitation. The therapist thanked her, and said all of the dishes and toys would be there next week when she came.

The following week, at the fifth visit, Mr. Lopez came to the office with his wife and Bonita. Bonita did not cry but sat very close to her father during the first part of the meeting. Later she accompanied her mother to look at some toys, and finally she was able to explore some by herself as long as the therapist was very far away from her.

Bonita was slightly more verbal, although it was clear that her language resembled that of a much younger child. Mr. Lopez was worried that Bonita cried so much and seemed so unhappy. He felt there was something terribly wrong with her "disposition." The therapist then mentioned again that Bonita seemed extremely sensitive to separations and that she had experienced many of them. She inquired about the kinds of preparation they ordinarily gave her for such experiences. The parents readily acknowledged that although they spoke to Bonita to give her directions or to tell her to stop something, they seldom otherwise spoke to the child. The therapist suggested that, because Bonita was so sensitive to separations, it might help to begin to predict things for her and to give her lots of time to prepare. She said it could prove very useful to tell Bonita exactly what was going to happen: who would go where and who would come back and when. She added that it would also be important not to deceive her; deception might avoid difficulties in the moment but it would cost them many moments of trouble later on. Because Bonita would remember the deception, future explanations of coming events would not reassure her as she would not believe them. Some discussion ensued: Both parents seemed impressed by these ideas, and said they would make an effort to talk to Bonita more about what was going to happen. In addition, it was noted that Bonita's wariness and their inability to fool her showed that the child could understand and connect things. They appreciated this as an indication of her intelligence.

It was increasingly clear to the therapist that these parents seemed to have no unconscious need for Bonita's behavior to be perpetuated. Instead, they seemed genuinely eager to understand and to try to do whatever was suggested. Mr. and Mrs. Lopez did not resist the understanding the therapist offered. On the contrary, they could quickly and easily accept the therapist's picture of Bonita's experience and could empathize with how Bonita had been feeling. This behavior strongly suggested that situational factors were the primary determinants of the difficulties in the parent–child relationship. In general, parent–infant relationship problems that have their roots in unresolved conflicts from the parents' own pasts are typically characterized by resulting negative attributions to the child and by an inability of the parents to experience what the child experiences. The parents' perception of Bonita was clearly free of this source of distortion.

At the end of the session the therapist used the toy telephone to ask Bonita if she would like to pick up the toys, and Bonita helped. While they collected them, the therapist described how it would be when Bonita came next week, who would come, and what they would do. She said that Bonita would be "in charge."

For the next weekly visit, as in the first home visit, only Mrs. Lopez and Bonita were present. The baby was at home with Mrs. Rodriguez. Bonita had been ill the night before, and she seemed very tired. This time her mother very readily allowed Bonita to determine when she would be on her mother's lap and when she would explore the toys. Mrs. Lopez was very excited that when she had told Bonita the night before that they would be coming to the playroom today, Bonita had begun playing with the phone. Also, in the morning Bonita had gone to select a dress to wear, whereas usually there would be a battle when Mrs. Lopez wanted to dress Bonita in order to go outside. The therapist said she thought it helped Bonita to have a feeling of control over things. Mrs. Lopez replied that she and her husband were making a great effort to explain things to Bonita. She also said Bonita had interacted a little bit more with other children in the household and had not been as isolated. The therapist and Mrs. Lopez then discussed the importance of not pushing Bonita but giving her time to "catch up." During this visit Bonita was much freer in exploring both the playroom and the waiting room. When she left, she paused near the therapist and said, "Bye."

The next session was Bonita's fourth visit to the playroom. It began with Bonita walking unhesitatingly with her mother toward the therapist and smiling. The change was striking and dramatic. She immediately approached the toys and began by playing with the telephone. She brought toys to both her mother and the therapist and engaged with the therapist in a game of peek-a-boo from beneath the table—giggling for the first time. The therapist could be responsive to Bonita's initiations now without frightening her, and Mrs. Lopez began "playing" with Bonita from across the room, verbally commenting and joining her in an exploration of toys. Bonita was now able to interact comfortably with her mother across this distance—apparently experiencing the mother's mere presence as comforting and reassuring instead of needing to touch her.

The quality of the mother–child interaction had shifted markedly. Mrs. Lopez would call out to Bonita about a toy she had and tell her how smart she was to have found it. Bonita would turn to her mother and hold up a toy, and her mother would smile and comment on how nice it was. This ability to experience a connectedness across physical space seemed to the therapist to bespeak Bonita's new internalization of the comforting nurturant and protective qualities of her mother which had been lost at the time when the pair were first observed. This change also allowed Mrs. Lopez to interact with her daughter in a way which totally satisfied Bonita but relieved her mother of the burden of clinging and demanding physical contact. Mrs. Lopez reported that Bonita was welcoming some very modest interaction with the other woman in the household. She said that preparing Bonita seemed to make a great difference, and she and her husband were being very careful to do this. Mrs. Lopez was very pleased with the changes that were occurring. When Bonita showed signs of fatigue and came near her mother whining slightly, the therapist suggested that perhaps they should heed Bonita's signal and end the session—suggesting that Bonita was tired and ready to go. The mother readily agreed.

The fifth session needed to be in a different playroom, and Bonita responded to the change by inspecting the new room thoroughly and unhesitatingly. She was pleased to find all of the familiar toys, and began playing with them contentedly. Mrs. Lopez, the therapist suddenly realized, looked ten years younger and significantly more relaxed. She reported that when she had told Bonita the night before that she was coming to the office, Bonita had gone to the phone again and said, "Hello, hello" a number of times. In the morning she had looked in the closet to choose a dress for herself and then had spontaneously looked through her baby sister's things and found clothing for her—wanting her to come. Mrs. Lopez had told Bonita that next time they would bring Cecelia. Mrs. Lopez was delighted as Bonita seemed in general more attached to and affectionate toward the baby. This made Mrs. Lopez' time with the baby easier and more enjoyable.

Also, Mrs. Lopez said that Bonita was in general happier at home and interacted more positively and more frequently with all the members of the household, now allowing herself to be approached and even held. She had played a peek-a-boo game with Mrs. Rodriguez, and everyone had enjoyed it. Mrs. Lopez said that she would bring the baby next time because Bonita wanted her to come. She spoke of Bonita as "bright." She said she was nearly toilet trained and had begun imitating her mother in caring for her sister. Bonita would look for a diaper or a bottle when Cecelia cried, and would find and summon her mother. Bonita was distressed if her mother did not come quickly to comfort the baby. This amazed and delighted Mrs. Lopez.

During the session Mrs. Lopez spoke frequently to Bonita, and began to be able to split her attention comfortably between Bonita and the therapist. The therapist commented on her skill, and Mrs. Lopez smiled with pleasure. As they were leaving, Bonita approached the water fountain, indicating that she was thirsty. Without struggle or even hesitation, she readily accepted the therapist's offer to lift her up to drink.

On the sixth visit, Bonita ran to the therapist as she approached the playroom and offered her some colored sticks. Mrs. Lopez had brought Cecelia and told the therapist that Bonita had decided what Cecelia should wear. Bonita accepted the therapist's help in getting out of her raingear. She then directed the therapist to Cecelia while she ran into the playroom to the two toy telephones. Bonita had been playing with toys for some time but her attention to only one toy was limited. Also, although her verbalization was continuously increasing her speech remained both immature and difficult to understand. Still, there was gradual improvement in these areas.

The interaction among Bonita, her mother, Cecelia, and the therapist was complex but smooth. Mrs. Lopez was easily able to attend to her two children and the therapist, and again the therapist commented on how well Mrs. Lopez could take care of everyone. Mrs. Lopez said it was easier now that Bonita did not seem to want her attention continually and was really beginning to play.

Then Mrs. Lopez voiced her worry about a pediatric check-up scheduled for Bonita several weeks hence. Those visits were always such horrible experiences. Despite the changes in her daughter, Mrs. Lopez remained apprehensive about what the upcoming medical appointment might be like. The therapist suggested that, just as preparing

Bonita in general had proven very useful, it might be helpful to prepare her specifically for the visit with the doctor.
The therapist got the toy doctor kit out of the cabinet and
asked Bonita if she wanted to help open it. As soon as it
was open and Bonita saw some of the familiar items, she
became very uneasy and moved far away. The therapist
empathized with Bonita, saying she knew that Bonita saw
some things like this in her doctor's office and didn't like
them. She said that she would just leave the equipment
out for Bonita, and when she wanted to play with it she
could. Bonita maintained her distance for a very long time
but finally began playing with the blood pressure cuff.

Mrs. Lopez began discussing her unhappiness with
the lack of privacy in their living situation, and when Bonita approached her with a toy she failed to respond. Bonita flung herself on the floor and started to cry. The
therapist and Mrs. Lopez discussed Bonita's distress at being unnoticed by her mother and noted, as well, her
mother's somewhat distressed mood. They recalled the
time when Mrs. Lopez had been so lonely away from her
husband and so ill during her pregnancy, and how upset
Bonita had been as well. In the course of this conversation,
Mrs. Lopez comforted Bonita. Later Mrs. Lopez mentioned that she was weaning Bonita from the bottle, at
which Bonita, hearing her mother, demanded a bottle, was
refused, and again flung herself down on the floor. Her
mother said there was no bottle, but they would have lunch
when they left. Bonita stayed on the floor watching her
mother though she stopped crying. Bonita responded immediately to the therapist's offer that they pick up the toys
together, and the visit ended.

Bonita began the next session by immediately playing
with the now-familiar toys. Somewhat later she ap-
praoched the open doctor kit and then attempted to take
the therapist's blood pressure. Mrs. Lopez invited Bonita
to take her sister's blood pressure, which they did together.

Then Bonita asked her mother for her bottle. When her mother said there wasn't one but that they would have lunch when they got home, Bonita lay down on the floor and whimpered quietly.

In response to the therapist's questioning, Mrs. Lopez said that she and her husband disagreed about Bonita and her bottle. After Mrs. Lopez steadfastly refused to give Bonita a bottle all day, her husband came home and gave her one. When Mrs. Lopez got rid of Bonita's bottles, her husband had taken one of the baby's bottles to give to Bonita. Mrs. Lopez and the therapist discussed how important it was for Bonita to get consistent messages. Also, they agreed that a number of Mr. Lopez' ways of handling Bonita seemed designed to keep the child's expectations toward him as positive as possible. As Mrs. Lopez and the therapist talked, they could see that as Bonita's preference for her father was beginning to shift and her relationship with her mother was improving, Mr. Lopez might be missing his specialness a bit. It was important, though, to get an agreement between the parents so that Bonita could be protected. Each might have to give in a little to the other.

During this conversation, Bonita calmed herself, played happily with the toys, and rarely interrupted the conversation. Occasionally what was being discussed was restated for Bonita, but she remained primarily engrossed in the dishes, pots, and stove. She paid some attention to the doctor kit, as well.

At the next visit Bonita went directly to the doctor's kit and got the cuff to take her mother's and the therapist's blood pressure. She also used the stethoscope and listened to everyone's chest. Early in the session, Mrs. Lopez said that her husband was thinking of going to visit his parents in a couple of months. He would go either by himself or with Bonita and stay a month. Mrs. Lopez didn't want him to go and was also concerned as to what this would mean for Bonita. The ensuing discussion made very clear that

Mrs. Lopez had become aware of what separations had meant to Bonita and what they might still mean to her. She also included the new information that, during the last five months of her pregnancy, she had been told to spend most of her time in bed. She had complied with her doctor's orders and had rarely left her bed. The probability that Bonita had experienced this as yet another kind of dramatic "loss" of her mother was discussed. Most evident was how dramatically Mrs. Lopez had shifted from seeing Bonita's behavior as "bad temperament" to understanding that her behavior was explicable in terms of her experiences. At one point, when Mrs. Lopez voiced her concerns about her husband's going away alone, Bonita flung herself on the floor and had a tantrum. The connection was pointed out by the therapist, and the reassurance and understanding provided by both Mrs. Lopez and the therapist was sufficient to calm the child.

Mrs. Lopez was genuinely concerned about what this disruption in their routines and relationship might mean for Bonita and was determined to discuss the issue with her husband. Although Mr. Lopez had attended no further sessions, his wife had kept him well informed about the meetings, and, as Mrs. Lopez said, "He can see for himself how different Bonita is." Mrs. Lopez and her husband had continued to discuss the issue of Bonita's bottle, but now Mrs. Lopez expanded her concern. Mrs. Lopez not only continued to give Bonita a bottle, but he diapered her when he took her out. He placed her in her sister's infant seat when he worked on his car so she could watch him. Every day when he came home from work he brought her a present. Mrs. Lopez scolded him for "spoiling" Bonita, but Mr. Lopez replied, "She is still a baby." In response to this the therapist asked how Mr. Lopez was with the new baby, Cecelia. Mrs. Lopez replied that he was not really very interested in the baby, and the baby was not particularly interested in him. The therapist commented that Bonita, then, was the only baby he had—and one less exclusively his than she had been for many months. Mrs. Lopez responded to this by becoming very thoughtful. The therapist supported the need for Mr. and Mrs. Lopez to speak frankly in order to understand one another and to give Bonita a united and consistent set of expectations.

In the next session Mrs. Lopez joyfully reported a "good" discussion with her husband. The day before he had not given Bonita her bottle when he had come home from work but had substituted a long walk to the store for some chips. Bonita had been delighted. In fact, it had been clear to Mr. Lopez that this excursion was much more fun than simply giving Bonita a bottle. This led Mrs. Lopez to mention that they were both using substitution with Bonita instead of just yelling at her to stop some behavior; this was working very well. It was an approach that had been suggested and practiced in the sessions. In addition, Mrs. Lopez reported that Mr. Lopez had begun to show a great deal of increased interest in Cecelia following their discussion. This was being reciprocated by Cecelia. It seemed that if Mr. Lopez could give up his need for Bonita to be his "baby," he was able to turn his attention to Cecelia and to begin to enjoy her.

During the session Mrs. Lopez successfully set limits for Bonita a number of times, was aware of her success and of Bonita's good-natured response, and was very pleased. She saw Bonita's cooperation as evidence of her daughter's intelligence and ability to understand things. At one point, when Bonita had a friendly exchange with the therapist, Mrs. Lopez remarked that Bonita was quite friendly now with Mrs. Rodriguez. She said Bonita often continued to play at home what she had played at the office and reported again that Bonita's initial contacts with Mrs. Rodriguez had been around peek-a-boo, just after she had played peek-a-boo with the therapist. Mrs. Lopez was very interested in the therapist's description of peek-a-boo as a separation game at the level that a child could control and enjoy. As Bonita and her mother left, they played a chasing game initiated by Bonita. It culminated in Bonita's allowing herself to be caught. Both Mrs. Lopez and her daughter experienced a great deal of pleasure in this interaction.

Now during visits Bonita moved in and out of the discussion, played happily with a variety of toys, and progressed in her self-paced explorations of the doctor kit. She gave injections to everyone, including all of the dolls. Her mother had been telling her that she would be seeing the doctor soon, and Bonita frequently repeated this to her mother at home. She was now scheduled to see the doctor the next day; when told this by her mother she repeated the information.

At the next session, Mrs. Lopez gave a glowing account of the visit to the doctor. Dr. Forrest had been able to approach Bonita, examine her, and interact with her without any undue fuss. Everyone had been delighted. In fact Dr. Forrest had been so pleased that she independently called the therapist at the Infant–Parent Program to describe what she called "this transformation."

Consolidation

For the following three months, visits to the Infant–Parent Program continued. This period saw a consolidation of new approaches by the parents and continuing development by Bonita, as well as a focus on the family's discomfort in their current living situation. The difficulties Mrs. Lopez had experienced in defending herself against Mrs. Rodriguez' excessive expectations of help were addressed, and Mrs. Lopez became much more assertive. Mr. Lopez not only had postponed his trip until the entire family could go, but in addition, he was thoroughly enjoying his baby daughter and no longer seemed to need Bonita to be "his baby." As a final effort, the therapist spent time with Mrs. Lopez choosing an appropriate nursery school.

Bonita's expressive speech was greatly improved, though it continued to be somewhat immature and difficult to understand. The parents had some concern that Bonita might have a minor hearing loss, and a medical investigation of this had been initiated. Meanwhile the therapist helped Mrs. Lopez to make sure that she always captured Bonita's attention when she spoke to her. Otherwise, Bonita was functioning well in all areas. She played with enthusiasm, enjoyed interaction with a number of different people, and showed no signs of inexplicable mood shifts, tantrums, or hysterical crying. In fact, a decision to terminate was arrived at in part because Bonita began to prefer outings in the park to visits to the office.

Summary

This case demonstrates the efficacy of a relatively intensive but fairly brief intervention aimed at helping parents understand and appropriately respond to increasingly disturbing behavior. In this instance Bonita's growth had slowed to a halt around the time of her mother's pregnancy and the enforced dispersion of the family. From the time of the unhappy separation of Mr. and Mrs. Lopez and Bonita's loss of her father, through the loss of her mother's availability during pregnancy, and an actual separation when her mother was hospitalized for a week, Bonita's experiences had not been understood. Her loving, well-meaning parents became increasingly discouraged and unwittingly handled her behaviors in ways which exacerbated them. Mrs. Lopez reacted to the loss of her agreeable and pleasant child with hurt and anger, which were then translated into rejection and distancing. Once reunited with his family, Mr. Lopez welcomed his child's dependence upon him and responded by infantilizing her during the time they spent together.

Neither parent evidenced any need for Bonita's behavior to persist as a way of expressing some internal conflicts of their own, however. Beyond this, neither had any impediments stemming from their own histories which stood in the way of nurturant relationships with their daughter. The difficulties between Bonita and her parents were primarily a result of situational factors. This made intervention considerably easier but no less critical. In the climate of misunderstanding surrounding the Lopez family at the time of referral, a spontaneous resolution was impossible. Bonita's behavior, which was not understood and was responded to unhelpfully, would only have become more disturbing, and the quality of family interaction could only deteriorate.

Timely intervention, however, enabled Bonita to change her current behavior dramatically and augured well for her continued good development. Both parents learned to understand and respond appropriately to Bonita and to collaborate more effectively with one another in their roles as parents. In addition they began to look for solutions in other areas of their lives which would work for the family as a whole.

References

Fraiberg, S., ed. (1980), *Infant Mental Health: The First Year of Life*. New York: Basic Books.

Lieberman, A. F. (1983), Infant–parent psychotherapy during pregnancy: A case illustration. In: *Infants and Parents: Clinical Case Reports*, ed. S. Provence. New York: International Universities Press.

———— Pawl, J. H. (1984), Searching for the best interests of the child: Intervention with an abusive mother and her toddler. *The Psychoanalytic Study of the Child*, 39:527–548. New Haven, CT: Yale University Press.

Pawl, J. H., & Pekarsky, J. H. (1983), Infant–parent psychotherapy: A family in crisis. In: *Infants and Parents: Clinical Case Reports*, ed. S. Provence. New York: International Universities Press.

7

Infant–Family Psychotherapy: One Approach to the Treatment of Infant and Family Disturbances

Chaya H. Roth, Ph.D., Margie Morrison, M.S.W.

Infant–Family Psychotherapy

Functioning in infancy, whether healthy or disturbed, is never a solo affair. Parents have the primary task of facilitating in their very young children the development of a personality structure, an experienced sense of self. The capacities of the self include: self-regulation; experiencing affect along all sensory modalities; fostering organized thinking and motoric adroitness; becoming attached

Acknowledgments: The authors gratefully acknowledge the support and contributions of the Irving B. Harris Foundation and the Jean and Walden Shaw Foundation, both of Chicago, Illinois, and Daniel X. Freedman, M.D. (former Chair of the Department of Psychiatry at the University of Chicago) which enabled us to establish and develop the work of the Parent–Infant Development Service. We are grateful, as well, to Bennett L. Leventhal, M.D., Director of the Child Psychiatry Clinic, for his unfailing support at every stage of our work. Finally, to the Jordans and to all of our patients, students, staff, and colleagues, including Zanvel Klein, Ph.D., who reviewed this paper with care, our thanks for their trust in us, their collaboration, their interest in our work, and their significant questions.

and caring; differentiating inside from outside phenomena, and self from others; communicating verbally and making mental and symbolic representations. Adherence to social mores and definition of gender identity, moreover, are also mediated by the experiences of the self with significant others (Sroufe, 1979; Greenspan, 1981). As the term is defined and used here, the *self* is the key to the formation of id, ego, and superego; it supplies these psychic structures with context, organization, and direction.

Just as the infant develops in the facilitating context of the parenting environment, so too do the parents continue to define and redefine themselves as a consequence of their interactions with their infant (Bell, 1968; Beckwith, 1972; Clarke-Stewart, 1973; Brazelton, Koslowski, and Main, 1974; Emde, 1981; Stern, 1977). Therefore, understanding normal and distorted development in the infant, the parents, and the infant–parent relationships depends on the amount and quality of useful information one can gather, process, and apply. In practical terms, this translates to the scope of the diagnostic evaluation, the diagnostician's knowledge of developmental norms and deviance throughout the life cycle, and the versatility and range of psychotherapeutic interventions available in any given intervention center.

In the Child Psychiatry Section of the University of Chicago's Department of Psychiatry, we have established a Parent–Infant Development Service (PIDS) that approaches infant and parenting problems from a broad biophysical, neuropsychological, and social–environmental perspective. We typically conduct comprehensive diagnostic evaluations that include medical examinations; neuropsychological assessments of infant functioning and temperament; evaluation of parenting functioning and parenting capabilities; evaluation of infant play; evaluation of parent–infant and family–infant interactions; and evaluation of the family's environment, living conditions, and social supports as perceived by the parents.

Assessment in PIDS starts with six to seven clinical interviews in the course of which the focus ranges over both the child and the parents. The topics are, in the main, what one would expect in a psychiatric clinic. The child's development is traced and current and past temperament are assessed. Later interviews cover each parent's familial history, development and current functioning, the nature of the marriage, the course of pregnancy and delivery, and the parents' reaction to the introduction of the baby into the family. The family's current social supports and the quality of their physical environment are also surveyed.

In addition, the child is seen in diagnostic play and for psychological testing. The child and parents are also observed and videotaped in a series of "set" situations. Each parent plays with the child in free play (3 minutes), teaches the child something new (3 minutes), and says goodbye, just as he or she might ordinarily do; leaves for sixty to ninety seconds and then reunites with the child (3 minutes total). The last "set task" (5 minutes) is that of the family having a snack together. (For a detailed description of the PIDS evaluation process, see Roth, Levin, Morrison, and Leventhal [submitted].)

Our extensive evaluation leads to an initial diagnostic profile of the infant–family unit. This profile helps in determining who participates in the treatment ("the strategy"), what the target of treatment should be to begin with, and what the emphasis of the treatment should be.

Psychotherapeutic approaches on behalf of infants and their parents involve a number of strategies and emphases, as well as the possibility of multiple, concurrent, or successive treatments. "Strategy" refers to the rationale involved regarding who participates in the treatment at any given time. For example, one parent will participate with the index child, both parents participate with the index child. Any individual member of the family alone, all significant family members together, both parents as a couple, and/or the siblings without their parents will participate. (Each of the treatment approaches is described in a monograph by Roth et al. [submitted].) The "emphasis" in approach refers to the technique and theoretical rationale of a given intervention. In our case, that means the degree to which psychodynamic, insight-oriented, and relational psychotherapy or didactic/problem-solving treatment and/or behavioral modification is used. We hold that many psychotherapeutic modalities involve all three aspects, in fact. However, depending on the developmental assessment of the particular patient's capabilities and goals for treatment, the emphasis may vary and, moreover, may shift over time.

We choose our emphases in terms of two primary criteria: (1) the nature of the infant's developmental dysfunction—an organic deficit is treated differently from a dysfunction rooted in a distortion of experience of expression; and (2) the nature of the parents' developmental character structure and organization, namely, their capacity to tolerate thinking, feeling, and working on behalf of the child without being unduly governed by their own infantile needs or deficits. Emphases may shift over the course of treatment as a result of gains by either the child or the parent(s). For example, didactic/problem-solving and behavioral techniques seem to be very useful in the initial phases of treating severe conduct or organically based dysfunction. However, once the parents achieve better control of themselves and of their children's behavior they may be ready to change from the initial emphasis on control, contingency, and reinforcement to a kind of therapy which is more introspective, experiential, genetic, and psychodynamic.

Infant–family psychotherapy is one of the intervention strategies developed by PIDS. Its uniqueness lies in the fact that the sessions include the infant and the parents, as well as siblings and other significant members within the nuclear family. Why have the infant there? A frequent rationale for this strategy is family or marital discord in which the infant has become the manifest object of the parents' or whole family's unhappiness. The future development and functioning of the infant may be jeopardized in such a circumstance. However, an important criterion for infant–family psychotherapy is that the infant, at the time of the evaluation, is not so seriously disturbed or delayed as to require the total and full attention of all present.

In infant–family psychotherapy, parents, siblings, and the infant (to the extent that the child is capable of it) reflect upon the meaning each has for the other, with a particular emphasis on the meaning of the infant. Issues of separateness and autonomy are usually triggered, as well as the matter of mutual dependence; these vary with the characterological development of each individual at the onset of treatment.

In a conflict-ridden marriage or family, the baby may become a vehicle for parental conflict. Each parent may seek the baby's exclusive loyalty, each may see their good or bad parts in the image of the baby, making it dangerous for the baby to get close to any one family member (for fear of alienating the others), and difficult for the baby to develop his or her own propensities. Family members react to the infant through the prism of their own experiences; they combine fragments of their "memories" with what the baby brings to a given situation. Infant–family therapy, moreover, explores the baby's capacity to evoke in the others powerful feelings that cannot be put into words. In the process of this exploration, the therapist and those in the family who are attuned to the baby's needs act as translators.

The presence of the baby draws infant–family psychotherapy to a level of communication different from that of traditional family therapy. The premium cannot be on symbolic fluency. To reach every member of the family unit, communication must be of a kind which includes the one least capable of symbolic representation (i.e., in most cases the infant). In practice, this involves "rephrasing" verbal messages and putting them in prelinguistic affective, cognitive, and physical form. The role of the therapist is multilingual, as it were. It resembles that of a translator who carries the message of the infant to the parent and the message of the parent to the infant, all the while teaching the "language" of the one to the other. Gradually, the interchange between the infant and the family members becomes direct. The therapist becomes less of a mediator and more of a resource person who interprets intentions and meanings when no one else can.

Transference interpretations, which form the crux of psychodynamically oriented treatment, require special expertise and differentiation. In family life, transference is what binds people in the family to one another. It represents what each individual sees in the other with which he or she already identifies or wishes to identify. Involving what each person likes or dislikes in him- or herself, the elements of transference in intrafamilial relationships are what each person will react to most strongly.

Since transferences in family life are already multiple, in the family treatment context transferences to the therapist are by and large not interpreted unless they threaten to disrupt the therapeutic alliance with the therapist.

This paper illustrates infant–family psychotherapy with one family in which marital conflict and individual parental pathology had threatened to compromise the development of a 15-month-old little boy. The strategy of the treatment was to include all three family members in most of the fourteen months of therapy. The emphasis of the treatment was primarily psychodynamic and interpersonal. While didactic problem-solving and behavioral modification certainly occurred and contributed to new learning, the primary task was understood to be exploratory. We used introspection and observation to clarify individual psychodynamics, interpersonal strivings, and identifications.

After summarizing our diagnostic evaluations, we present our analysis of the infant–family profile. The course of treatment in various phases is described next, followed by a discussion of the psychodynamic, interpersonal, and systemic principles that inform our approach to infant–family work. Finally, the paper ends with an outcome evaluation of our case illustration.

The Jordans

Self-referred, the Jordans were an intact, white, middle-class family consisting of a once-divorced 34-year-old father, a 30-year-old mother, and their first-born son, 15-month-old Bobby.

The Jordans' initial focus of concern over the telephone was Bobby: they were worried that he was too independent for his age and insufficiently affectionate toward them. They also alluded to marital conflict since Bobby's birth.

By the time of their first diagnostic interview, they were no longer particularly concerned about Bobby. Their marriage was now the problem. Mr. Jordan had left his job as a railroad dispatcher two weeks after Bobby was born and had been unable to find a new position immediately. His wife had to return to work as a secretary, therefore, less than four weeks after the delivery. Mr. Jordan became Bobby's primary caregiver. After seven months at home, Mr. Jordan got another job with a different railroad, but on the night shift. His work schedule let him remain at home with Bobby during the day, but prevented any sustained contact with Mrs. Jordan except on weekends. Moreover, soon after the conception of Bobby, all sexual activity between Mr. and Mrs. Jordan had ceased.

Needless to say, this was not a simple marital problem. From the very start, it was clear that Bobby had been an integral part of his parents' problems virtually since the day he was conceived. We decided to proceed with a comprehensive family diagnostic evaluation so as to better understand their distress; the Jordans agreed.

The following section is a summary of our diagnostic evaluations of the three members of the Jordan family, the relationships within the family, and the family's social–environmental context. The data include our first impressions, personal histories of the individuals in the family, psychological test findings, and clinical ratings distilled from interviews, clinical observations, and the videotaped interaction paradigm.

THE INDIVIDUALS IN THE FAMILY

First Impressions. Bobby was a beautiful child whose very appearance captured the attention of onlookers in the halls and waiting room of our clinic. His striking blond hair and blue eyes set off very fair skin and beautifully round facial features. To add some spice to it all, he showed a hint of mischief in his smile. His physique was sturdy and his gait solid and determined.

At first, Bobby was somewhat hesitant about being in a new place and needed his parents' encouragement to enter the doorway of the office. Once inside, he hovered close to his parents for a few minutes and then freely explored the objects in the room. He handled the toys competently and appeared well coordinated. Every once in a while, Bobby would bring a toy to one of his parents, seemingly anticipating the positive reaction he indeed received. He carefully observed Ms. M, the diagnostician (she was later also to be the therapist), and responded cooperatively to her efforts to engage him. However, he did not initiate contact with her until the next session when he generously included her in his game of depositing toys in the laps of all three adults in the room.

Bobby's receptive language seemed excellent. He responded well to directions, both in his ability to understand a request and in his enjoyment at carrying it out. This usually involved picking something up and either bringing it to a specified parent or placing it on the table. He vocalized frequently; an occasional word was intelligible. After a few visits to the clinic, Bobby was familiar enough to begin using "no" when he wanted to assert himself.

Bobby often sought physical closeness with both of his parents. He molded to both mother and father when held, but seemed to prefer active play on the floor with the toys. When he accidentally bumped his head or leg on the office furniture, he immediately turned to one of his parents for consolation. Though both were sought out to comfort him, Bobby approached his mother on that score more often than he did his father.

Bobby seemed to have a good sense of his own frustration tolerance and attention span. Toward the end of every session (which coincided with his usual nap time), just as he was becoming irritable, he would point to his bottle and ask for "juice." He then sat or lay on the floor, contentedly sucking his bottle for the remainder of the interview.

As the sessions proceeded, Mr. and Mrs. Jordan felt increasingly comfortable in talking about their marital problems. Bobby reacted to the sound and feel of the emerging hostility by banging toys against the wall. We surmised that he was attempting to distract and disrupt the conversation and, at the same time, to communicate his own level of discomfort. This little boy was clearly a "doer" who had no intention of allowing the events in his world to proceed without his active participation and influence.

Mrs. Jordan was another attractive member of the family. Like Bobby, she was fair in complexion and hair color. She also had pleasantly round and symmetrical facial features. However, her appearance was sometimes marred by skin blemishes at the sides of her cheeks. Often, these were a barometer of both her emotional tone in the session and the tension level at home over the previous week.

Initially nervous in the intake session, Mrs. Jordan spoke softly and appeared somewhat constricted. As she warmed up, her voice rose. She then became more articulate and began using gestures. After some hesitancy, it was not long before she became engrossed in describing her husband's faults, particularly her perception of him as irresponsible, weak, and vain. She spoke with conviction, but appeared frightened of offending him.

At times her eyes would begin to tear, but she would quickly pull herself together, seemingly upset at her loss of composure. Mrs. Jordan did not allow herself to feel sad for more than a moment. "I don't want to talk about it and I won't," she would often say. She cried later during therapy, but still could not tolerate permitting her husband, her child, or the therapist to witness her tears. On several different occasions, she simply fled the office.

Whenever Mr. Jordan spoke of his own inadequacies or tried to explain his side of a quarrel, Mrs. Jordan listened attentively, yet rarely responded with understanding for his viewpoint. As she saw it, in fact, every time Mr. Jordan faltered in his responsibility to her or the family, it was an indication that he did not care for them enough.

Although it seemed that Mrs. Jordan met every one of her husband's advances with an iron shield, her occasional tearfulness invited his closeness. A T-shirt she sometimes wore dramatized the invitation even more. The skin-tight shirt which accentuated her bustiness, read: "Eat Your Heart Out, I'm Married."

Mrs. Jordan's softness and warmth came through in her relationship with Bobby. She usually had a special smile reserved for him and very willingly followed his lead in play.

Mr. Jordan was a handsome older version of his son. He was immaculately dressed and seemed to take pride in his appearance. However, as he himself noted, he lacked the affability his son projected so easily. Mr. Jordan thought that this was due to his own limited self-confidence; in this respect, he was overtly envious of Bobby. Very articulate, his intelligence and insightfulness were evident as he spoke. Nonetheless, there was a sense that Mr. Jordan was continuously checking himself and that he relied heavily on the confirmation of others.

Mr. Jordan appeared to be almost begging for his wife's attention and respect. When she contradicted him, he characteristically backed off and acted hurt or humiliated. When he raised his voice in an infrequent manifestation of anger, he hastily retreated into an apology. (Both Mr. and Mrs. Jordan appeared frightened of strong expressions of emotion.)

With regard to Bobby, Mr. Jordan showed delight and pride. He beamed at him and followed his son's every move with adoring wonder. On occasion, he spoke firmly, even with a hint of harshness at Bobby's refusal to cooperate immediately, yet in the next instant he would envelop his son in a warm embrace.

It was clear that Mr. Jordan had a tremendous investment in Bobby, that he liked his wife, and that he was strongly motivated to work at improving their family life.

History. Bobby was a full-term baby born after what mother described as an uncomfortable pregnancy. The forceps delivery was uncomplicated, and Bobby weighed in at 6 pounds 10 ounces. Mother and baby left the hospital after four days and settled in comfortably at home.

Both parents were delighted with their son and perceived him as appealing, approachable, and easy to care for. In responding to items on the Bates Infant Temperament Scale, each parent independently characterized Bobby as easier-than-average to comfort and to predict and as average in activity level and adaptability to new situations and people. By his parents' reckoning, Bobby was mild in temperament and responded positively to their coos and smiles. He felt cuddly and molded well to both parents; each remembered that eye contact with him as a small baby had always been good. In addition, Bobby was a well-regulated baby. He fell asleep quickly and slept soundly. He was bottle-fed on demand, but generally conformed to a four-hour schedule as a young infant. Never colicky, he also welcomed with gusto the introduction of solid foods. Both parents related with pride that as Bobby grew older, he maintained his pattern of good eating and sleeping. He rarely protested having to nap and could usually amuse himself for quite a while in his crib before calling for his parents.

Bobby's health had been generally excellent, except for a time around three months of age when he had a persistent cold and sore throat. He never had any real difficulties with elimination; when he was occasionally constipated, he reacted well to the addition of fruit to his diet. Toilet training was planned to begin at around age 2. Mr. and Mrs. Jordan were prepared with potty seat and gum ball machine, although they were uncertain as to the details.

Bobby's developmental milestones were all within normal limits. He turned over at 5 months, sat unattended at

8 months, crawled at 9 months, and walked alone at 10 months. He was well coordinated and competent at both gross and fine-motor tasks.

Bobby had always been a vocal baby, imitating and producing sounds; at the time of the evaluation, he jabbered and spoke a few words. He had said his first word ("hot") at around one year of age. At 15 months, during the course of his diagnostic evaluation, he could also say "Mama," "Dada," "no," and "juice." As noted earlier, both parents felt that Bobby usually understood them when they spoke to him; he indeed demonstrated an excellent receptive vocabulary during visits to our clinic. Scores on the Bayley Scales corroborated the parents' report and our clinical observations. Bobby's MDI of 97 and PDI of 98 indicated that mental and motor development were within average limits.

The parents identified stranger anxiety in Bobby between 7 to 8 months. By 10 or 11 months of age, separation anxiety was at its peak. Bobby became most upset when he perceived that his parents were going out on a weekend evening. At 15 months, he would greet his neighborhood teenage baby-sitter at the door with a smile, but began to cry as soon as he saw his parents putting on their coats to leave. He tended to cry until his parents were out of sight and then was easily consoled and engaged in play by the baby-sitter. Bobby had no identifiable transitional object, but his parents related that he often requested a bottle just as he became cranky and usually sucked his thumb for short intervals prior to bed and nap time.

Mr. and Mrs. Jordan occasionally disagreed about setting limits for Bobby. Sometimes Mrs. Jordan felt that her husband "forgets [Bobby] is a little baby" and that he set expectations for propriety too high. More commonly, however, the complaints came from Mr. Jordan, who believed that his wife was too lenient in allowing Bobby to enter freely and play in their bedroom at night or by day.

Bobby enjoyed the company of both parents, but preferred different activities with each.

In short, Bobby was a healthy, active, engaging toddler who functioned age-appropriately in the physical, cognitive, emotional, verbal, and social realms. There were some indications of difficulties, however, in the areas of attachment to and separation from his parents.

Mrs. Jordan was the youngest of two children. Her brother, four years her senior, was married and had a 3-year-old son. Mrs. Jordan maintained frequent contact with her brother and sister-in-law and felt quite close to both. Her parents had divorced when she was 12 and her mother remarried several years later. (Four years before Bobby's birth, her father, living "no better than a bum," had died alone in a rooming house at age 56 of the ravages of alcoholism.) Although her mother and stepfather lived in the same metropolitan areas as Mrs. Jordan, she rarely saw them. Like her husband, she was distant from her extended family, but was supported comfortably by a network of friends.

Mrs. Jordan's childhood was extremely stressful. Her parents were in constant conflict, usually about her father's drinking. Although he held a job for several years, most of his paycheck was spent at the neighborhood bar. When Mrs. Jordan was 7, her mother was forced to go to work to support the family.

Despite her father's drinking, Mrs. Jordan felt that they had had a special relationship. She was "Daddy's girl" and remembered the family as she and her father versus her brother and mother. Mrs. Jordan felt that her mother preferred her brother over her and would always take his side in an argument; even when she was older, Mrs. Jordan believed that her mother never understood or supported her point of view.

After the divorce, Mrs. Jordan moved with her mother and brother to a new neighborhood.

In spite of initial difficulties in the new school in adjusting socially and doing the work, Mrs. Jordan mobilized herself. In high school, she made a few friends and began to date. She was, however, forever critical of her own appearance. Initially, she disliked her flat chest and skinny legs; as she developed, she was equally repelled by the fullness of her breasts and the roundness of her body. Her relationships with boys were fleeting: "Once I got the guy's class ring," she said, "I didn't want him anymore."

Another difficult period of Mrs. Jordan's life began when her mother remarried. Mrs. Jordan feared and despised her stepfather and was often involved in "horrible battles" with him (verbal ones). Much to her distress, her stepfather once made a pass at her; although enraged, she felt it would be futile to tell her mother. Upon graduation from high school, Mrs. Jordan moved out on her own. She held a number of successively higher-paying secretarial jobs, generally liked her work, and was competent and skillful at it.

Until she met her future husband (she was then 27 years old; he was married, but separated), Mrs. Jordan had had only one or two other significant dating relationships. Attracted to Mr. Jordan initially by his "good looks," she thought that he was "aloof and conceited." After his stormy divorce, the Jordans lived together for a short period and then married. Their romance rapidly cooled.

Before marriage, she and her husband had not discussed having children. Mrs. Jordan shocked her new husband when she declared that she wanted none for fear of becoming tied down and losing her sense of freedom. When, several months later, Mrs. Jordan became pregnant, the news came as a terrible blow to her and, she thought, to her husband as well.

Mrs. Jordan remembered three significant dreams during her pregnancy, all involving her giving birth under special circumstances. In one dream, she saw herself giving

birth as her mother lay dead in a nearby coffin, surrounded by mourners. In another dream, she gave birth
in a forest in the presence of her brother and some friends.
The third dream involved the baby being taken from her
before she could hold him.

Throughout her pregnancy, Mrs. Jordan felt depressed and moody. She experienced nausea on and off
for the entire nine months, in addition to constant heart-
burn and aching gums. She also had an episode of blacking
out. For a woman accustomed to excellent health, this period of debilitation was especially burdensome.

She also felt alienated from her husband throughout
the pregnancy. Initially, she said, she had withheld physical affection from him because of her anger at becoming
pregnant. Later, she assumed that Mr. Jordan had decided
to cease making love to her because he feared hurting
the baby; she had secretly wanted to continue their sexual
relationship but could not tell him. She complained that
her husband had shown no interest in going to prenatal
classes nor had he shared her excitement at first hearing
the baby's heart beat. After Bobby was born and Mr. Jordan had quit working, she was so enraged at him that she
"would have kicked him" had he approached her sexually.

Mrs. Jordan was in labor for eleven hours. Although
she had difficulty at times maintaining her Lamaze breath-
ing rhythms, she was proud of never having screamed.
Her husband, though uninvolved in the early stages of
pregnancy, had become a good coach and shared with her
the marvelous moment of birth.

It pleased her to have given birth to a boy because she
felt boys were easier to care for, were more obedient, and
not as easily hurt. At first, she had felt some guilt at "expecting a whole rush of love and affection for (Bobby)
which wasn't there." With time, however, the bond developed and she no longer worried.

Mrs. Jordan had strong convictions about raising her son differently from how she had been brought up. She intended to be firm—even "ground him" or slap his hands, if necessary—but, unlike her mother, she wanted to explain the reasons for punishments. She also hoped that Bobby would feel more free to talk with her than she had about talking with her mother.

It was Mrs. Jordan's wish that Bobby grow up a level-headed, confident, and happy child. She wanted him to have the ability "to walk into and master any profession he chose because he knows he's got our backing. I'm behind him if he's a doctor or a bum." In the long run, she hoped he would be "perfect." For herself, Mrs. Jordan aspired to a "life on Easy Street without having to rob from Peter to pay Paul." She wanted to be able to pay all her bills with ease and have money left over to buy presents.

She welcomed the challenge of treatment, though not without some ambivalence about having to share the work with two other people. As she said, she had always taken pride in doing things all by herself.

Mr. Jordan was the third of four children, all of whom still lived in the same city. His oldest sister, ten years older than he, was a recent widow and the mother of two children. His brother Tom, an aggressive entrepreneur, was seven years older than Mr. Jordan and divorced. His youngest brother, eight years Mr. Jordan's junior, had recently separated from his wife; he worked sporadically for Tom. His father had died two years before, at the age of 68. Mr. Jordan was not close to his extended family, but had a network of friends. However, his relations with authority figures at work was problematic—he persistently felt undermined and unappreciated.

In his early life, Mr. Jordan had been closer to his father than to his mother, although none of the family members were ever well-connected emotionally with one another. His father ruled the household and was never physically demonstrative toward any of the children. Because he considered his own thoughts and feelings as insignificant and unrespected by his father, Mr. Jordan developed a style of withholding his ideas and opinions.

Mr. Jordan's mother was a passive woman who kept to herself during much of his childhood. He recognized later that she too must have learned to hide her emotions, much as he had, because of his father's criticism. It seemed to Mr. Jordan that, as children, he and his siblings had taken advantage of their mother, rarely obeying her or considering her important.

For all his emphasis on getting ahead, the elder Mr. Jordan was a failure in the business world and never managed to make ends meet. Mr. Jordan saw his father as having lacked aggressiveness and self-confidence, qualities in which he viewed himself similarly wanting.

The person whom Mr. Jordan viewed as perhaps the most powerful childhood influence on him was his older brother, Tom. He was the hero whom Mr. Jordan admired for his fiery pugnacity and enterprising spirit, and whom he tried to emulate. Despite all his attempts to please Tom, Mr. Jordan believed that Tom had always disregarded and been inattentive to him.

Mr. Jordan felt positively about his years in grammar school where he was part of a large group of friends and was a good student. The change to high school was very hard. His parents had insisted that he attend an all-male high school; many of his friends went elsewhere. Although a "B" student and varsity athlete, Mr. Jordan was generally unhappy and lonely in high school. He often felt ostracized and rarely socialized.

Upon graduation, Mr. Jordan attended a university. After a year, he transferred to a junior college, where he found the atmosphere more relaxed and developed several good friends. He subsequently enlisted in the Navy.

After a two-year stint (he had been stationed in the South), Mr. Jordan returned to his home town and worked for a time at various jobs, mostly for Tom. On his own, he then landed a position as foreman of a new company. He was to spend the ensuing ten years climbing up the ladder of command with that company, though his relations with his bosses remained stormy.

Outside the work arena, Mr. Jordan was once again enjoying an active social life and dating. At age 25, after having had one serious romantic relationship and a few "inconsequential" ones, Mr. Jordan married an 18-year-old woman whom he had been dating for a year. He had been taken by her beauty and flattered by her attraction to him. The marriage lasted three years. Mr. Jordan acknowledged that he may have contributed to the break-up by forbidding his young wife to work; her alternative was to spend her time drinking in bars with her single girl friends. It was during the separation from his first wife that Mr. Jordan became interested in Mrs. Jordan, then a secretary in his firm.

Mr. Jordan saw the first year of his relationship with Mrs. Jordan as having been satisfying and pleasurable for both. By the time of the diagnostic, they were still affectionate with one another, but their sexual life was nonexistent. Worried about his performance and capacity to satisfy her before Bobby was conceived, Mr. Jordan completely relinquished sex thereafter.

The couple had discussed having children before the marriage; Mr. Jordan simply assumed that, like him, his wife would want children eventually. When she became pregnant (it was unplanned), neither he nor she would consider abortion, despite the unfortunate timing. In Mr. Jordan's mind, they were not financially ready for a baby. Since both parents felt strongly that a child should be raised in a house, they felt compelled to buy and move into one within a very brief period of time. Consequently, the financial pressures on them grew considerably just as Mr. Jordan was becoming increasingly dissatisfied with his job.

During the pregnancy, he perceived himself as unable to alleviate his wife's discomfort or boost her spirits. Mr. Jordan felt distant from his wife. He did not talk with her about his pleasure over the baby's prenatal development and his excitement upon first feeling the fetal heartbeat.

Both parents stayed home with Bobby for the first two weeks after birth. Then Mr. Jordan decided to quit his job, attributing his decision to a dislike for the work and a belief that he was not doing it well. It was seven months before Mr. Jordan found another position. To keep up the house payments, Mrs. Jordan went back to her old job. Mr. Jordan became Bobby's primary caregiver.

Although he said that he "took some offense at being a mother," Mr. Jordan conveyed a sense of great satisfaction and competence (his occasional uncertainties notwithstanding) at taking care of Bobby. The most gratifying aspect of parenting for Mr. Jordan was getting his son's affection. He also enjoyed feeling that much of what Bobby learned had come from him, although he saw Bobby as a joint reflection of his wife and himself. The most difficult part of being a father was disciplining the boy. Mr. Jordan did not like to hit Bobby but believed strongly that he needed to be more respectful. Occasionally, Mr. Jordan found himself unduly harsh with the child.

Mr. Jordan's aspirations for Bobby were for his son to realize early that he will "need to survive in the world out there." He felt keenly that Bobby ought not to have overly high expectations about what it would be like to be an adult. If his son learned discipline and received good schooling, Mr. Jordan believed Bobby would develop the ability to make his own decisions.

Mr. Jordan had high hopes for change as a consequence of treatment. He emphasized that this was the first time in his life that he had decided to put some effort into handling his problems.

The Assessment Profiles. As mentioned earlier, our extensive clinical data collection on each family member is reduced at the end of the diagnostic period to an assessment profile (see Table 7.1). For the sake of the text of this paper, however, the detailed profiles on all three members of the Jordan family are overly cumbersome and thus superfluous. The full-scale version of the profile is presented, for the sake of illustration, only in the case of Bobby's individual functioning; for Mrs. Jordan and Mr. Jordan, we have settled for briefer summaries.

Based on the information derived from the interviews, the play and testing sessions and videotaped parent–child and family interactions, we evaluated Bobby's functioning along five developmental "lines" (affect, cognition, physical-motor patterning, social relatedness, and language) and on his mastery of certain developmental "tasks" (homeostasis, attachment, somatopsychological differentiation, behavioral organization and initiative, and mental representation) as delineated by Greenspan (1981).[1]

Developmental Lines

Affect—3: Bobby's demonstrations of emotion had a wide and appropriate range as well as intensity. There hovered about Bobby, however, a mild vigilance that was a sign at least of concern, if not anxiety. His facial expression was generally one of interest with a mildly

---

[1]The ratings, based on a consensus of clinicians, range from 1 to 5: 1 = exceptionally adaptive; 2 = adaptive; 3 = marginally adaptive, 4 = maladaptive; and 5 = severely maladaptive (See Table 7.1. For a full description of the scales and their derivations, see Roth et al., submitted.)

TABLE 7.1
Bobby's and Mr. & Mrs. Jordan's Profile of Clinical
Assessments at Intake (T₁) and After 14 Months of
Treatment (T₂), by Context of Functioning

I. INDIVIDUAL CONTEXT

Areas of Assessment	BOBBY T_1/T_2	MOTHER T_2/T_2	FATHER T_1/T_2
Developmental Lines[a]			
Affect	3/2	3/2	3/2
Cognition	2/2	2/2	2/2
Physical Motor	1/1	2/2	2/2
Social	3/2	2/2	3/2
Language	2/2	2/2	2/2
Developmental Tasks[a]			
Homeostasis	1/1		
Attachment	3/2		
Somatopsychological Differentiation	2/2		
Behavioral Organization, Initiative	2/2		
Mental Representation	3/2		
Psychological Differentiation	NA/2		
Consolidation	NA/NA		

LEGEND:
[a] 1-5 Scale (All Lines, Tasks, Issues)
1 = exceptionally adaptive
2 = adaptive
3 = marginal
4 = maladaptive
5 = severely maladaptive

serious touch. He conveyed his enjoyment of activities, toys, and people by smiling, laughing, and jabbering; he communicated refusal and resistance in his distinct and determined "no."

Cognition—2: Capable of imitating actions, following directions, and negotiating goal-oriented and "permanence" tasks, Bobby demonstrated cognitive competence within normal limits for his age. He had a good sense of time, space, and the concept of at least the

TABLE 7.1 (*Continued*)

I. INDIVIDUAL CONTEXT

Areas of Assessment	BOBBY T_1/T_2	MOTHER T_1/T_2	FATHER T_1/T_2
Developmental Structural Schema[b]			
Ego Defects			
Defects in Self–Object Representation			
Major Constrictions			
Moderate Constrictions			5/4
Encapsulated Disorder		3/	
Adaptive with Phase Conflict		/2	
Adaptive with Flexibility			

Bayley Scores			
MDI	97/		
PDI	98/		
Stanford-Binet			
IQ	/103		

DSM-III		*Mo/Fa* T_1/T_2	
Axis I[c]	V61.20/None	V61.10/None 300.40/None	
		Fa	
Axis II[c]		301.60/in remission	
Axis III			
Axis IV[d]	4/3	5/2	5/3
Axis V[e]	4/2	4/2	5/3

LEGEND:
[b]1–10 Scale (Developmental Structural Schema)
1 = adaptive
2 = adaptive with phase conflict
3 = encapsulated disorder
4–5 = moderate constriction
6–7 = major constriction
8–9 = defects in self–object representation
10 = ego defects

LEGEND:
[c]DSM-III Classification
V61.20 = parent-child problem
V61.10 = marital problem
300.40 = dysthymic disorder
301.60 = dependent personality

LEGEND:
[d]1–6 Scale (Psychosocial Stressors)
1 = none
2 = minimal
3 = mild
4 = moderate
5 = severe
6 = extreme

LEGEND:
[e]1–7 Scale (Highest Level of Adaptive Functioning)
1 = superior
2 = very good
3 = good
4 = fair
5 = poor
6 = very poor
7 = grossly impaired

TABLE 1 (*Continued*)

II. FAMILY CONTEXT

Areas of Assessment	Mox I T_1/T_2	Fax I T_1/T_2	Areas of Assessment	IXMoxFa T_1/T_2
P-I Issues[a]			Infant-Family Issues[a]	
Initial Regulation	2/2	2/2	Availability	3/2
Reciprocal Exchange	3/2	2/2	Communication	3/2
Initiative	3/2	2/2	Problem Solving	3/2
Focalization	3/2	2/2	Routines	3/2
Self-Assertiveness	2/2	3/2	Goals	2/2
Recognition	3/2	3/2	Alliances	4/2
Dyadic Fit[a]			Marital Issues[a]	MoxFa
Availability	3/2	2/2	Availability	4/2
Reciprocity	3/2	2/2	Communication	4/2
Joint Activity	3/2	2/2	Problem Solving	4/2
			Routines	3/2
			Goals	3/2

Parenting Tasks[a]	Mo	Fa
Safety	2/2	2/2
Security	3/2	2/2
Nurturance	2/2	2/2
Appealing Environment	3/2	2/2
Play	3/2	2/2
Containment	2/2	3/2
Planfulness	2/2	2/2
Internal Representn.	3/2	3/2

LEGEND:
[a]1–5 Scale (All Lines, Tasks, Issues)
1 = exceptionally adaptive
2 = adaptive
3 = marginal
4 = maladaptive
5 = severely maladaptive

number "one." He knew body parts and could make means–end connections. He easily found objects hidden under cups, indicating retrieval memory. At times he did not persist at a task. The issue seemed one of a relatively brief attention span.

TABLE 1 *(Continued)*

III. SOCIAL/ENVIRONMENTAL CONTEXT

Areas of Assessment	*IxMoxFa* T_1/T_2		
Social Supports[a]			
Availability	2/2		
Quality	3/2		
Living Conditions[a]			
Economic	3/2		
Health	1/1		
Educational	2/2		
Home Environment	3/2		
Psychosocial Stressors[d]	*I* T_1/T_2	*Mo* T_1/T_2	*Fa* T_1/T_2
DSM-III, Axis IV	4/3	5/3	5/3

LEGEND:
  [a]1–5 Scale (All Lines, Tasks, Issues)
  1 = exceptionally adaptive
  2 = adaptive
  3 = marginal
  4 = maladaptive
  5 = severely maladaptive

LEGEND:
  [d]1–6 Scale (Psychosocial Stressors)
  1 = none
  2 = minimal
  3 = mild
  4 = moderate
  5 = severe
  6 = extreme

Physical–motor patterning—1: Bobby was particularly agile. His gait was smooth, sturdy, and well balanced, and he was adept at running. With ease, he executed tasks requiring fine-motor movements, such as building a block tower or completing a simple puzzle.

Social relatedness—3: Bobby tended to engage his parents easily and initiated a variety of activities with them, from playing telephone to playing ball. He clearly anticipated a positive reception from both his mother and father and always got it. It was typical of him, however, to make good contact, and then just leave. The abrupt leave-taking happened when each parent was alone with Bobby as well as when he was together with the two of them. After his mother or father had responded to him, he would at times walk off toward some unclear destination, leaving his mother or father to play with what he had brought to them. Often he would move toward the door; at other times, he just moved to another part of the room, roaming or looking for something else.

With Ms. M and the psychologist, after Bobby had shown initial and appropriate hesitation, he soon became engaged and, for the most part, was able to sustain the interaction.

Language—2: Bobby was vocal, jabbered frequently, had single words and short phrases in his vocabulary, and also gestured expressively to communicate his intentions. He had a relatively good understanding, as well, of what was said to him.

On the Bayley Scales he achieved an MDI of 97 and a PDI of 98.

Developmental Tasks

Homeostasis—1: Bobby was highly alert and attentive to his surroundings and was apparently well regulated. His emotional expressions were clear and distinct. He actively sought comfort when needed, but could also console himself.

Attachment—3: Bobby showed "primary attachment" to both his mother and father, displaying a marked preference for either parent over other people. In play, he related to each parent with appropriate affect and level of activity, but seemed more vigorous with his father. Nevertheless, his tendency to initiate games and then move away from one parent to look for the other was indicative of vigilance in relation to them and expressive of an undefined anxiety.

Somatopsychological differentiation—2: Bobby communicated and responded adeptly, using many sensorimotor modalities and showing a wide range of affect. Assertive and purposeful in his actions, he demonstrated a growing awareness of his ability to affect the outcome of an interchange or activity.

Behavioral organization and initiative—2: Bobby's actions were goal-directed and intentional. His determination in executing a task or conveying a wish was notable, but he could comply, after some protest, with the imposition of limits and structure.

Mental representation—3: Admittedly, Bobby had barely entered the phase of development during which he would come to rely on symbolic representation in social contexts. Still, the tenuousness of his play activities and the vagueness of his interests in toys were inconsistent with his generally well-structured awareness of his environment. It was thought that his anxiety might interfere in the development of concentration and thematic play.

DSM-III Diagnosis. Based on our initial evaluation, Bobby was given the following DSM-III diagnoses on Axes I to V (American Psychiatric Association, 1980):

Axis I: V61.20: Parent–child problem.
Axis II: None.
Axis III: None.
Axis IV: 4 (Moderate).
Axis V: 3 (Good).

Emotionally, Mrs. Jordan was slow to warm up; affect was constricted with prevailing feelings of sadness and anger. Intellectually, she appeared to be of at least average intelligence, showing good learning capacities in school, and good organizational capacities at work and at home. She appeared to be physically somewhat tight and restricted initially, but her posture was steadfast and she was well coordinated in her movements. In social interactions, she was reticent, moderately withholding, and somewhat rigid. Mrs. Jordan's communications were fluent and clear. On the Greenspan–Polk developmental ego-structuralization scale, Mrs. Jordan was assessed to have a capacity for a limited representational system and an encapsulated disorder of the self. This implies phase-appropriate negotiation of the early tasks of self-regulation, the formation of human relationships, differentiation of internal and external experience, organization of behavior, imitation and internalization, and representational differentiation. Her capacity to work and to relate to peers or superiors on the job was excellent. She experienced difficulties in gender identification and was conflicted about her womanliness.

Parenting Tasks. Mrs. Jordan provided safety and security for Bobby, as well as adequate nurturance in a matter-of-fact atmosphere with a moderate amount of tenderness. She also provided him with an appealing environment of playthings, including herself—she was always willing to play with him, but was not always sure that he wanted to play with her. As a result, she showed a certain apprehensiveness in play with Bobby. Mrs. Jordan set appropriate limits, containing her son as needed, but not unduly so. She helped Bobby anticipate events by preparing him for what was to occur; she also aided his postponing certain activities until all was in readiness. She did not feel sufficiently self-assured to convey to Bobby that she expected him to remember her admonitions when she was not with him. In this regard, she seemed to be tentative and emotionally removed.

Mr. Jordan showed a full range of emotions, though he was not always appropriate in the modulation of his emotional reactions (he was often overly diffident, critical, harsh, or self-depreciating). Of above average intelligence, he showed his intellectual skills in his academic achievements. His job performance was compromised by interpersonal conflict, not by his capacities to understand or perform the task. Physically, Mr. Jordan moved easily and well. When anxious he appeared constricted and not as smooth. In social interactions he tended to be ill at ease. Occasionally, he exploded in a fit of rage. He had no close friends and encountered much strife with authority figures. He communicated easily and clearly.

On the Greenspan–Polk developmental structuralization scale he was assessed to have moderate constrictions in ego structure, with limitations and alterations in the experience of affects and pleasure orientation, and severe impairment in self-esteem. Gender identification was impaired, as was his capacity to adhere to socially expected standards.

Mr. Jordan was conscientious and vigilant about safety and security. He nurtured his son with exquisite care, providing food in an optimally tender and solicitous atmosphere. He created an appealing environment for his son as regards toys and objects, as well as in his own enthusiasm at being with Bobby. In play, Mr. Jordan was equally enthusiastic and absorbed. As regards helping Bobby to be disciplined and contained, Mr. Jordan seemed overly concerned; he was therefore quick to anger when his son stepped out of line. Mr. Jordan emphasized the need to share, wait his turn, and ask for things rather than take them. In this way, he helped promote an attitude of planfulness and a capacity to postpone or delay. Mr. Jordan was inordinately caring and concerned that Bobby remember his admonitions. As such, he too, like Mrs. Jordan, showed a certain apprehension as regards the lasting nature of his impact on the child.

RELATIONSHIPS WITHIN THE FAMILY

Mother and Bobby. In the free-play segment of the first parent–child diagnostic interaction, mother and Bobby presented not as two deeply attached beings, but as two acquaintances—interested, yet somewhat tentative and wary of one another. Mother kneeled on the floor with several toys before her: a toy phone, puzzle, and cookie monster. She beckoned toward Bobby and encouraged him to play with her. He walked toward her, picked a puzzle up from the floor and, handing it to her, continued on by with a look of mild interest–disinterest in both his mother and the puzzle. Mrs. Jordan tried to engage him, but did not know quite how, it seemed. She looked over her shoulder and followed him as he moved past her and toward the door. There he stopped. He tried neither to open the door nor look under it. He just stood there and would not return to his mom. The free-play segment was definitely not a success for this pair.

At the next interaction segment, Teach-a-Task, however, mother was much less tentative and more ready to initiate and direct Bobby's activity. Given permission to structure his environment and impose her will on him, she came alive. Bobby responded, even if briefly, and when he refused to put the shapes in the box with a clear and adamant "No!," mother brightened. "No?" she said. "Okay. Do it your way then!" There was real pleasure in her reply. It seemed to us that she was less interested in a tower being built or getting the blocks in a shape sorter than in her son's accentuated response to her and his determination to do it his own way.

The separation sequence, which included leave taking, Bobby's remaining alone in the room, and reunion, proved to be very difficult for both mother and child. Mrs. Jordan left Bobby with but the barest of preparation, muttering inaudibly under her breath that she would return very soon. Bobby was inconsolably upset at his mother's leaving. He stood by the door and cried continuously. He stopped only momentarily to check out the noise which came from the revolving video camera on the ceiling and then resumed his position by the door in tears. These were three very long minutes for Bobby. And yet, upon mother's return, Bobby barely moved toward her. For her part, mother did not inquire about how he was feeling nor how he had managed without her; she merely tried to engage him in play, but her son passed her by once again.

Father and Bobby. The interactions between father and son were marked by frequent approaches toward one another. Each anticipated a positive reception from the other and both were usually rewarded in kind. Nevertheless, in the free-play segment, Bobby walked toward the door several times, as if he thought that someone was outside (though he did not seem to expect that anyone would be coming in). Mr. Jordan was not discouraged by his son's distance. He called him back engagingly: "Come here, Bobby, come on over here and see what I have. Oh! so you don't like the cookie monster? Well, then, look at his phone!" Sure enough, Bobby went over to play with it. He and his father then handed the phone back-and-forth making believe they were talking to someone on the other line.

In the Teach-a-Task segment, however, when Bobby asserted himself and refused to read a book with his dad, Mr. Jordan had trouble accepting his son's refusal and looked clearly displeased. It seemed that father had no trouble accepting Bobby's neediness or dependence but he did not care at all for his son's self-assertiveness and oppositionalism, though both were decidedly mild.

The separation sequence with father was markedly different from that with mother. Mr. Jordan's leave taking was long on preparation. He explained that he would be gone for only a very little while and presented Bobby with toys with which he could play in the meantime. Bobby's reaction to the separation was the same he had shown with his mother: he cried unconsolably and did not move from the door until his father returned. The reunion of father and son was warm on both sides: father immediately took Bobby in his arms, sat him on his lap, rubbing his stomach gently, and tenderly spoke to him about how hard it had been to remain alone without mommy or daddy.

Bobby and Family. The ambience of the family snack-time (the final segment of our video paradigm) was of disjointed relatedness. Father and mother neither looked at nor spoke to one another. They busied themselves with preparing for the snack: one opened the juice cans while the other arranged the crackers on the plate. Mother had chosen to sit across from Bobby (this was a rectangular table), leaving father the seat between her and her son. Consequently, Mr. Jordan ended up helping Bobby with his cheese and crackers. While father was putting the cheese on the cracker, his appreciative "Mmm! mmmm!" in a sing-song voice was repeated and imitated by Bobby with the same pitch and intonation. Mrs. Jordan just watched; her face expressed neutrality and a certain distance. On occasion, Bobby glanced at his mother furtively, but not long enough to sustain a possible response. Once, he offered her a cracker, leaning over from across the table, and extending his arm as far as it could reach. Mother was not to be engaged. "No, Bobby," she said, "This is for you; you eat it." She then withdrew further into herself, resting her head on one of her palms and looking on. Bobby resumed the sing-song dialogue with his father, but never completely ceased glancing over toward his mother.

Marital Relationship. Whatever the discordance in the infant–family relationship, the greatest tension rested without a doubt in the marital relationship itself. We knew of this from clinical observation, as well as by the Jordans' own reports. We have no video paradigm for parents alone and did not think fast enough to create one for the sake of this family. Nevertheless, what we had on videotape was ample evidence of Mr. and Mrs. Jordans' lack of communication. When they worked in concert, it was for the sake of Bobby; at that, their collaboration was primarily parallel. At home, in their new lives as parents, they decidedly parted ways. Their divergent work schedules precluded marital interaction. Just as Bobby had passed mother by in the free-play sequence, Mr. and Mrs. Jordan seem to pass each other by in their daily lives. Together only on weekends, they filled their time with household chores. One parent stayed with Bobby while the other ran errands. Communication was, at best, frigid and so was their sexual life—frozen out. When problems arose, they retreated further into their silence. On occasion, a loud thunderous explosion occurred between them; the subsequent withdrawal from one another seemed even more foreboding than before. The goals they shared in common had to do with Bobby's education, such as saving for good private schools. They were planning for his entering preschool at age 2 to 2½ and, with kindergarten, his beginning parochial school.

SOCIAL SUPPORTS AND LIVING CONDITIONS

The Jordan family had a group of friends with whom they enjoyed socializing regularly, particularly for weekend dinners out and a couples' bowling league. They could turn to their friends for baby-sitting on short notice and could borrow things from them in a pinch. Their extended families were available to the Jordans in an emergency, but the relationships with their families of origin were uneasy. Although old tensions had subsided some, they still surfaced from time to time. As a result, neither Mr. nor Mrs.

Jordan felt comfortable openly sharing their current dif-ficulties with their families. They felt they could not be understood.

A middle-class family, with their own home and two cars, the Jordans were not underprivileged, and yet, they did experience financial strain. Mr. Jordan's period of un-employment had ended with his subsequent shift to night work. Nevertheless, there was a continued necessity for his wife to remain employed to meet the family's new standard of living.

All family members were in excellent health, and had regular medical check-ups and excellent health insurance coverage.

Mr. Jordan had two years of college and was an avid reader. Mrs. Jordan's training had prepared her very well for her position as an executive secretary. Both parents maintained a strong investment in learning and education.

The Jordans owned their own two-story brick bunga-low. After Bobby's birth, Mr. Jordan had worked at re-modeling the attic into a separate room and play area for his son. By their account, the home was well-furnished, clean, and equipped with the kinds of appliances and en-tertainment devices which make a house physically com-fortable. Despite these material comforts, the Jordans ex-perienced their home environment as fraught with tension and therefore not a source of security or emotional warmth.

Summary of the Assessment Profiles. The Infant–Family Assessment Profile rated consensually by four members of the team, reflected our clinical understanding of the Jor-dan family (see Table 7.1).

Bobby's individual functioning was viewed as adaptive on most lines and tasks except for the marginal ratings on emotional, social functioning, attachment, and mental representation. As separate persons, Mr. and Mrs. Jordan were functioning only marginally or moderately maladaptively. The ratings also showed some marginal functioning in the quality of the interaction of each parent with Bobby. The marital relationship was assessed to be clearly maladaptive. Overshadowed by serious marital dissension, the family relationship was also compromised. Social supports and living conditions, on the other hand, were only marginally affected: The Jordans' relationships suffered from a lack of intimacy and their financial status and home environment were experienced as moderately stressful.

Formulation

Mr. and Mrs. Jordan came to PIDS because they believed that their marital difficulties not only reflected their own troubles, but were also creating problems for their child. They did not understand, though, how their marital problems had come to be or how they were being played out between them and in what ways they affected Bobby.

In the first years of their marriage, Mr. and Mrs. Jordan had struck a certain balance with one another. Each had complemented the other's needs: Mrs. Jordan gave her husband the nurturance and acceptance, as well as the narcissistic gratification, he had craved. Mr. Jordan gave Mrs. Jordan the feeling of being a married, loved, and attractive woman. At the same time, each was free to pursue his or her own aspirations—Mrs. Jordan's needs to show her continuing self-sufficiency and competence and Mr. Jordan's ongoing search for self-satisfaction in the masculine role.

The pregnancy changed things. It unsettled Mr. Jordan by bringing into sharper awareness his intense conflict over female–male identification. It placed on his shoulders a heavier burden of responsibility for effective performance on the job and within the family. Mrs. Jordan also reacted strongly to the pregnancy. She too had not wanted the pregnancy, but she was not undone by the prospect of motherhood. In a sense, she welcomed the opportunity to become the "full" woman she believed her mother to be. Her dreams reflected strong competitiveness with her mother and an intense wish to be admired. Moreover, by giving birth to a boy, she hoped finally to acquire the "maleness" and thereby the love that had been reserved only for her brother.

From the time of Bobby's conception, the relationship between the Jordans had gradually developed into a silent, sexual stand-off. With the birth of their baby, the family's balance was totally upset. Mr. Jordan's insecurity around assuming the masculine role on the job and the envy he felt toward his wife, led to his leaving his job and assuming the role of the boy's primary nurturer. Fathering provided Mr. Jordan with the pleasures of nurturing and valuing his son that he wished had been his lot when he was growing up. The problem for Mr. Jordan and Bobby was Mr. Jordan's extreme overidentification with his son. Projecting his own needs onto the baby and attempting to gratify himself by gratifying the boy, Mr. Jordan accentuated even more his anxiety over his masculinity. This, in turn, stimulated his projection onto Bobby of weakness of character—hence, the sharp reaction to Bobby's mild provocativeness. Enmeshed as he was in his own regression, Mr. Jordan as unable to assume his family responsibilities or to maintain his ordinary social ties. And, finally, he came to feel totally unfit for maintaining a sexual relationship with his wife. He was too depreciated.

For Mrs. Jordan, being with her husband during their preparenthood days had represented a double victory: on the one hand, she had won the affection of an attractive, giving male; on the other, since her husband shared her father's weaknesses, Mrs. Jordan could emulate her mother and even outdo her by being a better wife than her mother had been.

The birth of the baby and her husband's joblessness made Mrs. Jordan repeat her mother's hardship and robbed her of the joys of mothering and womanhood. While she identified with her mother, Mrs. Jordan had not felt fully affirmed by her. She had shared responsibilities with her mother, not love. The love Mrs. Jordan had wanted to receive without reservation went to her brother. Mrs. Jordan, even as a child, had been the "competence machine." As such, despite her wish to nurture and love, she behaved in her relationship with her newborn son the only way she knew. For him she became the publicly competent parent (going out to work to feed the family), not the intimate caregiver. With the birth of Bobby, her husband became more like her father and she, more like her mother.

For Mrs. Jordan, the lack of pleasure in being a loved and loving woman–mother was a deep-seated source of pain. In giving birth to a son, she had hoped to complete the identification with her mother and, at the same time, capture her mother's love by identifying with the boy she had produced. This theme was reflected in her first dream. She had seen herself giving birth to a boy—but felt *alone*, since her mother was dead in a coffin. In her second dream, Mrs. Jordan exposed herself by giving birth to a son in the presence of her brother and his friends. This represented the fulfillment of the wish to be admired as a woman—something she felt had been withheld from her.

Characterologically, Mrs. Jordan was the more developed of the two parents. Ego structure was well defined, but attended by painful affect (the loved self was devalued). For Mr. Jordan, on the other hand, ego structure was less cohesive. He had been more traumatized. His self-definition as a man had suffered and he grew up to feel insufficiently valued and competent. He searched painfully for an ego ideal. There were also lacunae in superego structure, as well as latent homosexual stirrings, passivity, and a chronic quest for dependent gratification.

Whatever the characterological problems and depressive signs in both Mr. and Mrs. Jordan, the nurturing of Bobby held a salutary and healing promise for each. Both needed to parent Bobby in order to restore to themselves what they had failed to get during their childhood. As a result, Bobby was moderately well nurtured and well parented but he was saddled with a huge task: namely, to be bridge and buffer for his parents and to satisfy their unassuaged childhood needs.

Bobby, for his part, while functioning within normal limits, was showing signs of hypervigilance, fear of separation, and too much random and unfocused activity. He did not and could not understand the nature of his parents' conflict but could sense that he served both of them in mysterious ways. Unless something changed, Bobby was at-risk for continued distractibility and a brand of pseudo-independence which could become the forerunners of an emotional and behavioral disturbance.

The Course of Infant–Family Psychotherapy

On finishing the diagnostic evaluation, we recommended infant–family treatment to the Jordans, therapy which involved regularly meeting with the two parents and Bobby together. We were led to choose that form of intervention because we believed the problems of the family to be not only in the marital relationship but also in the meaning that Bobby had for each parent, and in the Jordans' use of Bobby in their marital relationship. As such we thought Bobby's development was at risk. We were also struck by the Jordans' sensitivity and their capacity to work psychologically in spite of the intensity of their pain.

We believed that the presence of Bobby in the sessions would:

1. Highlight and keep in focus the meaning of this child to each of the parents;
2. Bring to the fore (more rapidly than if another modality was used) unresolved infantile issues within the parents that were interfering with their capacity to "parent" each other and indirectly were triggering anxiety in Bobby;
3. Attenuate the parents' natural resistance to experiencing and understanding the source of their pain and generate, for the sake of the child, the courage and energy to change.

In this process, we believed that Bobby's moderate problems would also be resolved.

In deciding to treat the family in infant–family psychotherapy, we thought everyone would gain a better understanding of the complicated personal and family dynamics. It was our goal to help heal the rift between Mr. and Mrs. Jordan and to strengthen their mutual bonds. Bobby could no longer be expected to do all the work—both to maintain himself and to bind the parents to one another. In the course of the work, we hoped Mr. and Mrs. Jordan would benefit in a deeply personal way, as well. A shift in basic personality structure was part of our goals too.

We discussed our thinking with the Jordans and, together with them, reviewed their histories and looked at the videotapes. They concurred with our rationale for infant–family psychotherapy and accepted our recommendations.

Over the course of the next fourteen months, the family was seen once a week. Of the total of forty-one sessions, eight were with just the parental couple. What follows is a description of the content and process of treatment as it unfolded in what we can now see as five constituent phases:

Phase I. During the initial phase of family treatment (which lasted about two months), all three members of the Jordan family were present.

Early on, Mr. and Mrs. Jordan began directing to the therapist (rather than to each other) a list of complaints about the other spouse. Mrs. Jordan interpreted her husband's indecisiveness and failure to assume financial responsibility for his family as a way of overburdening her. She was particularly critical of his excessive drinking, which she saw as an indication of his selfishness. If he really cared about her, Mrs. Jordan maintained, her husband would change. It was hard for her to imagine that Mr. Jordan had problems of his own that had antedated his acquaintance with her. It frightened her to think of him as having personal troubles (i.e., as weak and vulnerable). While able to express anger at Mr. Jordan, she was somewhat timid and reticent in her relationship with the therapist—like her, a woman. This was evident not so much in what she said but in her posture, turned-inward position, and her not being able to sustain prolonged eye contact with the therapist. (This was particularly obvious during a very early session when she appeared with her well-developed figure molded by a T-shirt which read, "Eat Your Heart Out, I'm Married.")

Compared to his wife, Mr. Jordan was warmer, more forthcoming, tried to please and engaged the therapist longer and more meaningfully. After some initial hesitation and with encouragement by the therapist, Mr. Jordan conceded his difficulties in trusting himself. He also charged that whenever he did take a firm stand, he was undermined by Mrs. Jordan, particularly where Bobby was concerned. Mr. Jordan felt that Bobby should not be present for prolonged periods of time in their bedroom, for example. According to Mr. Jordan, even after he had clearly stated his wish for privacy, his wife repeatedly permitted Bobby to remain in their room. (At this point, the wish to be alone with his wife was not linked to specifically sexual interests.) He interpreted this at first as her lack of respect for him; later, he came to see it as Mrs. Jordan's way of maintaining her distance.

From the beginning, Bobby was keenly aware of the acute dissension between his mother and father. He was very active in the office, in an unfocused way, roaming from toy to toy and unable to settle down.

In one session, after the tension level had risen, Bobby climbed into the infant seat and began to suck his thumb. The therapist first took note of Bobby's random play. Then she reflected to him that he needed to sit in the baby chair. She mused out loud to Bobby and the parents: "I wonder why Bobby needs to be in the baby chair? Could it be, Bobby, that mommy and daddy's angry feelings make you worry and you feel very, very small and alone just now?"

The therapist, when speaking about any member of the family—including (and in particular) Bobby—always addressed that person directly.

Ms. M. then translated the same statement to the parents. "I think Bobby gets frightened when the two of you talk about angry feelings and then he feels alone and wants to be very, very small like a baby."

The therapist was noting here that what appeared to be Bobby's self-determination was in fact infantile anxiety and an expression of his sense of aloneness. At the same time, she was also modeling for Mr. and Mrs. Jordan how one observes feelings and responds to them.

In the beginning, each parent was surprised that their little boy was not only aware of their marital problems, but also reacted as he did. With time, each began to apply this form of observing not only to Bobby, but also to one another and to themselves. Mr. Jordan remarked that when he and his wife were angry at each other, they tended to withhold their feelings rather than express them directly. His wife would first stew and then snap critically; he would distance himself by staying in another room or watching TV. Ms. M. suggested that just as they were learning to label Bobby's feelings, they could also learn to identify their own. For a long time, they practiced in the sessions. Gradually, this kind of reflectiveness began to generalize to their home life as well.

During these early weeks, Bobby played with toys in a corner of the room, approaching one parent or the other on occasion, or retreated into the infant seat.

When Bobby became distressed, each parent responded to him in characteristic style. Mr. Jordan saw Bobby as helpless and dependent, the way he felt himself to be. He would scoop Bobby up on his lap and cuddle him, at times excessively, providing his little boy with the comfort and security he craved for himself. Mrs. Jordan's response to Bobby's distress, on the other hand, was to try fostering greater self-reliance in the child. She would ease him off her lap and attempt to direct his attention to a toy or activity. Gently, tactfully, but straightforwardly, the therapist shared her impressions with the parents. Despite their discomfort, the Jordans tolerated these observations of their behavior—their capacity to take in the therapist's thoughts was apparently enhanced by Bobby's presence in the room. They could see that he, too, was in pain. The relationship with the therapist drew both on the parents' love of Bobby and on their own desire for mending.

Phase II. The second phase of the family's treatment (covering about 4½ months) was characterized by an intensification of feelings expressed during the sessions.

The couple began sparring, openly fighting, or sullenly withdrawing from one another. They continued to address themselves to the therapist, seeking her out as ally or buffer. The therapist encouraged the parents to talk to each other and to respond to one another directly.

Bobby became increasingly unruly. He sometimes tantrummed coming down the hall or into the office and repeatedly banged on the radiator with blocks. Once again, the two parents did not respond in the same way. Mr. Jordan often snapped at his son in a harsh tone of voice; Mrs. Jordan either ignored Bobby or attempted to bribe him with a cookie or toy. Only when the therapist encouraged the parents to think about what Bobby was experiencing did they relent from their own quarrels and attempt to think about and feel for the child. Bobby's anxiety also triggered personal associations within the parents. On one occasion, as mother was able to attend to Bobby's worry over his parents' quarrels, she was reminded how, as a little girl, she had had to face her own parents' chronic bickering. She began to cry openly—feeling for Bobby had opened a path for Mrs. Jordan to feel for herself.

In time, Mrs. Jordan grew more apt to pick Bobby up and keep him on her lap and was more at ease in thinking about his fears, anger, and vulnerability. In relation to the therapist, she became accepting of support, responded to her warmly, looked at her appreciatively, and in general conveyed a sense that she now had an ally.

Mr. Jordan viewed his wife's progress with a mixture of pleasure and envy. Consistently doubting himself, he felt he had not made the strides in treatment that she had. He also began to feel more and more envious of the new softness and sensitivity that Mrs. Jordan was showing toward Bobby. But in relation to the therapist, a new reticence set in. He felt less attractive and now looked toward her less for support. He didn't have it coming, he felt. The therapist did not interpret this sense of defeat in relation to her. Instead, she reflected his feelings in relation to himself and his wife. Mr. Jordan absorbed the concern and held it there for a while—standing still, as it were.

Eventually he was able to acknowledge not only envy of but also desire for his wife.

Mrs. Jordan was surprised and very pleased to hear of her husband's desire for her. What she had previously interpreted as rejection she now began to understand as her husband's difficulty in approaching her. During the course of one particular session, when Mr. Jordan admitted to her how he craved her affection, she was touched to the point of tears and then fled from the room—for fear that her husband would approach her only out of pity. For his part, Mr. Jordan wanted to run after his wife but held himself back for fear of rebuff. It was the therapist who helped Mrs. Jordan to return to the session and listen to her husband's feelings. Although she could not yet permit herself actual physical closeness, she acknowledged her husband's needs indirectly: she told Bobby (who had begun clinging to her and clamoring for attention) that it was important for the two grown-ups to talk to each other first; later they would both listen to him. Bobby's response was immediate and gratifying. His agitation dissolved in front of their eyes as he calmly returned to play with his dump truck.

That session ushered in the third phase of the treatment (it, too, lasted about 4½ months).

Phase III. Interestingly, Bobby began to show a new and persistent interest in his mother's breasts. Mrs. Jordan, though quite uncomfortable about it, was reluctant to stop Bobby for fear of hurting his feelings. She also was identifying with Bobby's need for closeness and his curiosity about her, and she was allowing herself the luxury of gratification. In spite of her discomfort, Mrs. Jordan, haltingly at first, was able gradually to examine her feelings about her own sexuality and womanliness. Her needs and those of Bobby and her husband were slowly disentangled until, in one session, she told Bobby (who was once again fondling her chest) that she knew he wanted to be close to her but that her breasts were private and she did not want him to touch them.

Bobby's behavior was a tip-off that sex and sexual intimacy would be the theme of this phase of the treatment. Ms. M suggested that Bobby not attend the next several sessions, but it was several weeks before Mr. and Mrs. Jordan came in without their son. Their willingness to confront and approach each other followed another of Mrs. Jordan's flights from the office.

She had begun the session by expressing disappointment that her husband had not acknowledged a record album she had sent him. She began to cry and ran from the room. This time it was Mr. Jordan, rather than the therapist, who followed her out and got her to return. He listened attentively and encouraged her to talk about having risked but gotten no response. A mutual sharing of feelings followed. At the session's end, the two hugged one another (the first time in over a year) and agreed to meet for the next several times without Bobby.

In these sessions, both spoke about sexual yearnings and of their feelings about being man and woman. Mrs. Jordan thought herself undesirable to her husband, while Mr. Jordan admitted being anxious and at times panic-stricken about his capacity to perform sexually. Each spoke about their past memories of thwart and shame, guilt and fear. Mr. Jordan feared rejection and ridicule most of all. Mrs. Jordan worried about being found out and punished. They spoke of their relationship to one another.

In this middle phase of their treatment, then, the Jordans were heavily embroiled in disentangling the distortions that had crept into their lives. And sexual identity was a key issue for both. In spite of progress they were making, it was clear that an abstinence of sexual intimacy of over two years' duration would not be easily overcome.

With the encouragement of the therapist, both Mr. and Mrs. Jordan considered steps they would be willing to take toward intimacy. What emerged was a process of courtship that was poignant in its awkwardness—but a start. Mr. Jordan purchased a massage book and gave his wife back rubs. Mrs. Jordan suggested that they shower together, but wore a bathing suit the first time.

Phase IV. Bobby's return to the sessions marked the start of the next three months of treatment; this phase of the work began with a bang.

To start with, Bobby refused to leave the waiting room and had to be carried down the hall fussing, kicking, and screaming. Once in the office, he went straight to the toy area and began throwing toys all about him as he moaned, wailed, and raged in angry despair. To no avail did mother, father, and the therapist each say, in different words, that they understood how angry and upset Bobby was over his enforced and long absence from the sessions. Bobby's pain was too deep to be dispelled by reflection and interpretation alone. Time, repetition, and feeling with and for him were required to soothe his anguish. In the past, each parent used to turn to Bobby almost exclusively for affection; now, with his mother and father's renewed closeness with one another, Bobby feared that he was expendable. And, to compound the injury, even his therapist had apparently deserted him! He, therefore, vented his rage on all three.

Bobby's anger and hurt touched Mr. Jordan in a special way. Comparing himself to his son, it occurred to him that as a child he had never expressed that kind of anger toward his own domineering and critical father. Encouraged by her husband's example, Mrs. Jordan also spoke of the injustices she had endured as a child by having to be the "strong" one in her family. As she talked, she gradually realized that her mother's demands and her father's attempts at seduction were not attributable to "badness" within her. The problem had not been hers alone, but also that of her parents and their marriage. With a somewhat altered view of her past, she began to feel better about herself and gained a new ability to express her softer side.

Bobby was now nearing 2½. Both parents thought that it was important for his learning that he be in day care and associate with other children. The plans for school registered within Bobby and led to renewed worry and negativism on his part. At home, he smeared toothpaste on the walls and overturned the stereo speakers. In the office, he returned to the infant seat. This time, his parents, not Ms. M, spoke to him about having mixed feelings about going away from home to school. They wondered out loud if he felt he was being sent away and if he felt that he had to remain a baby to be loved. They also spoke about how much fun it would be going to school like the "big kids" and all the activities he would enjoy with them.

The family was now relating sensitively and thoughtfully. The therapist was intervening less frequently. Thoughts about Bobby's growing up went hand-in-hand with thoughts about termination from treatment.

Phase V. The discussion of termination plans marked the beginning of the final two months of treatment. The gains made by each family member were reconsidered. Mrs. Jordan continued to acknowledge feeling weak when she wished to be touched either physically or emotionally, but was much more able to give warmth as well as to receive it. Mr. Jordan could become angry when necessary and could set limits in a more even and less erratic manner than before. Bobby's mood in the sessions had become calmer and more focused. He let himself get more absorbed in play and was less vigilant.

Outside the treatment sessions, as well, Mrs. Jordan became overtly more giving and Mr. Jordan began to take greater risks. Their sexual intimacy increased. By the time the family had ended treatment, Mrs. Jordan was, in fact, two months pregnant. This time the pregnancy was welcomed equally by both parents. Neither, however, lost

sight of the effect the arrival of the new sibling would
have on Bobby. There was much thoughtful consideration
about what he might experience. Appropriate plans were
made to prepare Bobby for the birth of the baby.

Discussion

The story of the Jordans can be used to exemplify
some principles of both theory and of technique. In
searching to illuminate aspects of normal and deviant development and the interplay of psychodynamics—individual as well as interpersonal—with the processes of treatment, we have found explanatory value in five principles:

1. Transactionalism (Sameroff and Chandler, 1975; Sameroff and Harris, 1979; Sameroff, 1982);
2. Projective identification (Klein, 1946; Jaffe, 1968; Zinner and Shapiro, 1972);
3. Equifinality (von Bertalanffy, 1968);
4. The use of "natural" transferences; and
5. The bidirectionality of effects (Schafer, 1978, 1982;
   Spence, 1982).

In the following pages, we would like to explicate these
concepts and show how they apply to the work of
treatment.

Transactionalism. A transactional approach to family
functioning means that individual family members are not
viewed in isolation from the others. They are best understood as growing and developing in interaction with one
another and changing, in part, as a result of their interactions. Transactionalism is a systems theory principle of
sufficient strength to account for significant effects both
between and within individuals.

The Jordans' presenting request for our help was evidence, we think, of their intuitive understanding of the

impact of this mutual influence. At some level of awareness, they knew that their marital conflicts had led to
Bobby's difficulties. We agreed, but we went further. We
viewed their marital problems as deriving from the resi-
dues of their own histories—their own developmental difficulties—exacerbated and altered by the arrival of their
first-born son which, in turn, had significantly changed
their relationship to one another.

Current research and an extensive clinical literature
both richly document the effects on parental functioning
of the multiple interactions of the histories of each parent,
the characteristics of the child, and the nature of the marital relationship (Benedek, 1959, 1970; Jessner, Weigert,
and Foy, 1970; Lerner and Spanier, 1978; Belsky, 1979,
1981). Although no research systematically and empiri-
cally demonstrates Lidz's contention, our experience supports his view that (Lidz, 1976) partners in a marital relationship seek each other out in the hopes that the one will
help the other complete his or her sometimes difficult but
always unfinished psychological growing. While the search
for oneself in the other is with the goal of adaptation, the
sequelae of such an undertaking can also sometimes be
maladaptive. That, we believe, is what happened with the
Jordans.

Mr. Jordan had been drawn to his wife for her competence, adeptness, and seeming autonomy. He also responded very positively to her admiration of his masculine
looks and her sexual attraction for him. Not only did he
identify with her autonomous streak, but he also hoped to
locate in himself the masculinity and sexuality she had seen
in him. For her part, Mrs. Jordan had hoped that if her
husband found her desirable, she would indeed be vali-
dated in her femininity. Thus, remaining the competent
woman her mother had brought her up to be, she would
also finally also be the sexual love object she never had
been in the eyes of mother nor in those of her all-too-often

drunken father. Bobby, too, evoked in his mother and father deeply personal associations of both hope and conflict. We have learned how the baby evokes in most parents certain unresolved problematic or as yet "unfinished" issues carried over from childhood or adolescence into young adulthood–parenthood (Benedek, 1959, 1970; Fraiberg, Adelson, and Shapiro, 1975; Fraiberg, 1980). The matter becomes even more complicated when one realizes that the infant has a different impact on the father, the mother, and each of the siblings. Each individual in the family sees the infant from a uniquely personal perspective. As a result, the infant acts toward and reacts differently to each of these individuals. Withal, the infant's repertoire is limited by his or her developmental and constitutional capabilities. The young child's response patterns are relatively few, relatively uncomplicated, and relatively elemental.

Projective Identification. Projective identification, as defined by Klein (1946), Jaffe (1968), and Zinner and Shapiro (1972), is an activity of the ego which modifies an individual's perception of significant others and, as a result, modifies the individual's image of the self. The process underlying this mechanism is one of projection followed by identification. This is achieved when an individual has attributed aspects of him- or herself to a significant other, perceives or misperceives these in the other, and then attributes these externalized aspects to him- or herself.

Bobby assumed many roles for his parents: he was not only the object of their projections and identifications, but he served also as the conduit for their communications. At the same time, paradoxically, he was the buffer that kept them apart.

In Bobby's anxieties and needs, Mr. Jordan saw his own weakness and vulnerability. He hoped to protect

Bobby from the fear of rejection by being particularly nurturing and caring for him. By doing this for Bobby he was, of course, also making restitution to himself. By giving to Bobby, Mr. Jordan was giving himself what he had never gotten and had only observed in others—his brother, for example. (We will have more to say about the restitution concept later in the discussion.) At the same time, Mr. Jordan could not help but become intensely sharp and angry with Bobby when he thought he had discerned in his son's behavior evidence for a possible "weakness" of character, such as his disobedience in following directions or his willfulness.

For Mrs. Jordan, Bobby was the culmination to her achieving a sense of womanhood. She had sought this much earlier in relation to her mother and father, but she had been only partially successful: Her mother had rewarded her only for performing household chores and other such responsibilities. She could not feel or show love and admiration for her own daughter and have the gratification of finding her own reflection in her. Presumably, Mrs. Jordan's mother had herself not experienced that in her own background. Mrs. Jordan had witnessed that kind of love, however; it had been showered on her brother. Her father's love and admiration were probably not too well received, since most of the time he was deemed to be unreliable. It is also possible that sometimes he was too forward with Mrs. Jordan, and, to protect herself from his advances and her own impulses, she had to keep him at a considerable distance. First her husband and then Bobby, therefore, provided Mrs. Jordan with a second chance for positive feminine feelings.

She was not to be allowed to luxuriate in this sense of victory for long, however. By giving up his job, Mr. Jordan forced his wife to fall back onto her old coping strategies, namely, to emphasize competence in the working world.

He thereby had taken away, as it were, her opportunity to gratify her need for intimacy and mothering.

Transactionalism from the systems perspective and projective identification from the psychodynamic, personal, and interpersonal perspectives help us understand a great deal about the interrelationships among various aspects of the individual, as well as about the impact that people have on one another. However, these two concepts cannot account for the enormous impact of the presymbolic child on those with whom he or she interacts. Of particular interest here is the uncanny power of the communications of the very young child (from soon after birth to about 24 to 30 months of age).

Anyone entering a room in which a baby is present, particularly if the baby is "doing" something, knows how everyone's attention gravitates to the child. A baby can keep several adults and older children spellbound, as they watch his or her every move and expression. What gives an infant's communications such force for the symbolically functioning person?

The power of the infant's communications lies in the very fact that they are not directly understood. They are experienced, we think, in part within an archaic, presymbolic mode that survives and remains active in everyone throughout the life span. The infant's expressions evoke presymbolic "memories," sensations, fragments of thought, and visual images that do not follow rational and logical syntax. Whatever the words we have to describe our experience as a result of an infant's communication, we are transmuting necessarily from one mode of experiencing to another; in the process, we will have captured only some, not all, of the infant's experience. What we were unable to translate into representational symbols and feelings resonates wordlessly within us and ignites almost ineffable fragments of experience. For these reasons, we are sometimes caught off-balance and always fascinated by the communications of the presymbolic child.

How then does one deal with such content—unmanageable in conventional language, yet so evocative? The mechanism involves another contribution of general systems theory, namely the principle of equifinality (von Bertalanffy, 1968).

Equifinality. Equifinality rests on the assumption that development is goal-directed and that there are multiple pathways leading to a developmental goal. Adaptation can occur along any number of paths, in a compensatory manner. Namely, when one avenue is blocked, development will nevertheless proceed along another route. Sometimes the compensatory path is opened naturally, without outside intervention. At other times, the route must be cleared or stimulated to enable the organism or system to assume the needed function.

Equifinality, then, clarifies for us that understanding another person's experience can be achieved through modes other than symbolic communication, for example. In most cases, this happens intuitively between babies and their caregivers, but where communication or understanding is blocked due to the emotional blindspots of the individuals involved, the therapist can serve the function of opening up blocked channels. Furthermore, we believe, alternative modes of understanding and communicating can be taught, first by modeling and second by explaining what one has modeled.

In most families, most of the time, one or all members can apprehend the infant's communications at all levels—symbolic, experientially affective, and even fragmented. One "feels" as if one has "understood" the baby—that he or she is uncomfortable, tired, frightened, wants to play, is bored, wants to be held, or wants to be put down, for example. One isn't always right, but even in error things proceed with a certain graceful flow. One observes the baby and then responds to it with a question or a tilt of the head. Perhaps one then shakes one's head and starts all over again, indicating, as it were: "No, that's not it. Maybe after all you need a little more of that or a little less of the other." Through trial-and-error one attempts through gradual approximations to enter into the inner experience of another being who hasn't the words or the concepts to convey the experience to us. Some have compared this flow between the senses and fragments of logic to the interplay which exists between lovers wherein symbolic language is but a part, sometimes a suspended part, of a larger totality (Sander, 1983; Stern, 1983).

There are, of course, occasions when the child's rage, pain, discomfort, helplessness, fear, or even the need to be held closely come to dominate the interaction, but cannot be assuaged, because they are "misunderstood." At those times, people around the infant can react with discomfort, impatience, oversolicitousness, loss of interest, or outright rejection. Where this kind of misunderstanding occurs repeatedly, both infant and parents tend to redouble their initial reactions. The consequence is spiraling and mounting distress on both their parts. Over time, such gross and frequent misunderstandings produce parents and babies who approach each other with a negative expectation—a false connection as it were—which is tantamount to a negative transference reaction. For these families, someone is needed to rebuild the bridge.

Sensitive to and tolerant of what he or she understands or merely senses, the infant–family therapist translates for the parents and others from one experiential mode into another. The therapist attempts to clarify and facilitate the translation of infantile experiences into the symbolic mode and thus enables others to appreciate the preconceptual. Conversely, the therapist also translates to the infant, at the level of the infant's capacity for understanding, the nature of the parents' distress. That is done both by inflection of the voice and by carefully choosing one's (simple) words. It is not the words, however, that convey the meaning as much as the melody which accompanies them.

This is accomplished first and foremost, through a particular kind of observation, which we have called "receptive" or "interested." Observation of that quality is indispensable to convey the availability of one person to another. The next step is that of conveying what one has observed. It can be done through mirroring, labeling, enlarging upon, infering or interpreting. (The details of therapeutic communication and its various steps deserve another monograph. We are currently at work on such a paper.) The words and intonation that the therapist uses in "translating" these expressions of another's experience are of the utmost importance.

The process of observing and conveying the meaning of the child's experiences to the parents and the parents' experiences to the child has been well illustrated, we think, in the description of our work with the Jordans.

From the very beginning, the therapist had encouraged the Jordans to observe their child's and their own experiences carefully. She had spoken directly to Bobby during the sessions—never "about" him, as if he were not present. When she did explain something about how Bobby was feeling or what he might be thinking, she first conveyed these thoughts to Bobby in his language, simply and directly. She then turned to the parents and translated these simple messages into adult parlance. The therapist had allowed herself to wonder out loud about what it was that concerned Bobby and she checked these thoughts with Bobby in trial-and-error fashion, slowly and clearly. All the while, she was explaining to the parents exactly what it was she was doing, hoping that in this manner the parents would begin to learn her technique.

The therapist's task had thus been threefold: (1) to understand the child's state much as she attempted to understand the state of the parents; (2) to show how she herself went about the business of understanding (i.e., to document, as it were, the intuitive process and how one approaches another's state of mind by gradual approximations); and (3) to "teach" these steps to the parents. The effect of this threefold process is a close approximation, we believe, of what Winnicott (1958) meant when he spoke of the therapeutic process as "creating a space within oneself" for another or, as we like to put it, to think and feel on the other's turf. Thinking on behalf of another person—or on the other person's turf—is what many authors have defined as "empathy" or "the empathic process" (see Buie [1981] and Basch [1983] for excellent summaries, and Kohut [1959], for an attempt at a seminal definition).

But equifinality, in itself—no more than transactionalism or projective identification—has insufficient explanatory power to account for *how* infant–family therapy heals both the parents and the baby. An account for the psychological change must invoke two additional and interrelated principles: (1) transference, and (2) the bidirectionality of effects.

Transference. We distinguish, in our work, between therapist-dominated and natural transferences. Therapist-dominated transferences are engendered by the treatment situation. In infant–family treatment, as in all forms of psychodynamics and psychoanalytically oriented therapy, the transference experience with the therapist is part and parcel of the healing process. The relationship to the therapist, in this context, assumes a special significance and everything else becomes a backdrop to it. "Natural" transferences develop without special prompting in the ordinary course of family life. Only in part projections and projective identifications, these transferences can also become manifest in disavowals, denials, reaction formations toward, and idealizations of one individual's perceptions, expectations, experiences, and wishes vis-à-vis any other family member. They are as powerful, if not more so, than those arising within the context of the psychotherapeutic relationship. Rooted in the day-to-day events and the history of the family, they do not have the "artificiality" of the therapist-induced transference. They do not have to be defended against and are thus ready to be addressed; therapist-dominated transferences, on the other hand, have to be developed first, are then defended against, and finally can be dealt with.

In infant–family psychotherapy, the transference manifestations are many: from each family member to the other—from parents to child, and from parent to parent. The therapist in infant–family work attends to these transference manifestations, reflects them empathically (thereby allying him- or herself temporarily with the person manifesting them), and helps clarify and disentangle them, thereby becoming a transference object in his or her own right (Fraiberg et al., 1975). As we practice it, however, in infant–family treatment, therapist-dominated transference is rarely interpreted. Since the therapist is an adjunct to anyone who is subject to or object of the natural transference distortions, his or her focusing on therapist-dominated transference would fragment the work, lead away from the dynamics of the family, and divert the goals of the family's treatment. Therapist-dominated transference manifestations are interpreted only when the therapeutic alliance per se is threatened—either within the family as a whole or with one or more individual family members.

Let us see how the analysis of the various kinds of transferences can be applied to the case of the Jordan family. Natural transferences were evident in the relationship of the parents to one another and to their baby. Mrs.

Jordan saw in her husband character traits similar to those she had observed in her father. She had been attracted to Mr. Jordan much as she had been to her father. Mr. Jordan had been the "forbidden fruit" (while married to another woman), but she nevertheless (or therefore?) had enjoyed his company. We believe that Mrs. Jordan's experience as "Daddy's girl" had a similar forbidden quality.

After she conceived, Mr. Jordan no longer wanted to make love to her. Feeling rejected, she attributed her husband's withdrawal to her undesirability. Without a solidly internalized sense of her femininity, Mrs. Jordan became depressed. After Bobby was born and her husband left his job, Mrs. Jordan felt driven to resume the managerial position which both she and her mother had assumed in her childhood years. She reverted to seeing her husband as the deficient, unmasculine provider her father had been. In Bobby, Mrs. Jordan saw both good and bad possibilities. Viewing him as the male she had produced, she both loved him more and valued herself more. When, however, he was less than enthusiastic with her in play, she felt immediately rejected as she had in the past (presumably in relation to her mother and brother).

In an idealized manner, Mr. Jordan saw in his wife what he would have wished his mother had been. He had married a much younger and less imposing woman the first time, presumably because he had to be sure his rather tenuous sense of virility was up to the task of being a husband. The woman proved too infantile and nonresponsive to his needs. Mrs. Jordan provided a much richer source for his further growth. Furthermore, her attraction to him was enormously flattering. When his wife conceived, Mr. Jordan's own unfulfilled infantile wishes surged to the fore. He began to regard his wife as an unapproachable, rejecting mother with other children to love. He was no longer able to perform sexually. When Bobby was born, Mr. Jordan completely relinquished all pretense at having to function in the adult male world. His son had come to represent his own babyhood. Through a process of identification, Mr. Jordan became at one and the same time his own and his son's major caregiver. Only in his son's bids at assertiveness did Mr. Jordan recapture some of his maleness (which he had internalized in partial identification with the men in his family). As a result of viewing Bobby's autonomy as a threat to his masculinity, he was capable of becoming overly harsh and punitive with his son.

What of Bobby? Can we say that he, too, experienced natural transference feelings toward his parents? Probably not. From a developmental and theoretical perspective, it makes little sense to posit that children and adolescents have natural transference feelings toward their own parents. They can, however, experience them toward older or younger siblings, parent-substitutes, and/or any other individual who is not their primary caregiver.

And what of therapist-dominated transference? There were many, of course.

In the beginning of treatment, Mrs. Jordan had been intimidated by her woman therapist with whom she compared herself most unfavorably. Her single, rather feeble shot was the implicit boasting about the size of her chest (her T-shirt reading "Eat Your Heart Out") but she then shrank into her seat for the rest of one of the early therapy sessions, totally unable to address the therapist. Much of Mrs. Jordan's reticence in the early sessions was due to a negative transferential attitude. It was deliberately not addressed, however. Instead, the therapist reflected (and reflected on) Mrs. Jordan's need for positive feminine confirmation. Only after she came to understand the origins of this need and developed a very positive and trusting attitude toward her therapist did Mrs. Jordan dare to divulge her hesitations, her fears of being found unacceptable, and her need for being admired and loved. The therapist was the transference catalyst, but the transference had remained uninterpreted.

Mr. Jordan started in quite a different way. He was seductive toward the therapist, tried to please, and was cooperative in all ways. As the truth of his married life became more obvious to him, he became quieter, sullen, and depressed. There was a sense of defeat in the air. It was never clear whether the defeat was felt in relation to the therapist or to his wife, but the therapist did not press forward with a transference sally. In fact, she encouraged the theme of defeat to develop in relation to the wife, not to herself. With Mrs. Jordan, he was involved in a natural transference with a history, ongoing life experiences, and a future; that was the relationship to work with, and they did.

The one person in the Jordan family whose transferential relationship with the therapist was emphasized was Bobby. As he was with his mother, Bobby was tentative with the therapist and not quite fully engaged. He looked at her only furtively and went back to his play. He roamed from toy to toy and was unable to settle on any one in particular. He searched for father's affection and avoided mother, even as he avoided the therapist. When he became angry, he vented some of the anger at the therapist. After an interruption of treatment for him—when only his parents came—Bobby, upon his return to the session, poured his outrage upon the therapist. She responded to every one of his communications, verbal or nonverbal. She reflected his general feelings and, in particular, his reactions to her, the latter with the same emphasis as she placed on his reactions toward his parents.

Given the significance of transference phenomena, natural and therapist-dominated, how does dealing with transference restore the individual to a higher-level and more adaptive way of functioning?

A possible explanation for the change rests with what we have termed the principle of the bidirectionality of effects.

Bidirectionality of Effects. Though the term is ours, the basic concept belongs to systems theory since it addresses changes that occur inter- and intrasystemically without reference to unconscious forces or defense mechanisms, but rather to the realm of communication and its effects.

The principle reflects the views of Schafer (1978, 1982) and Spence (1982) according to whom experiences in the present which are transference manifestations of the past, when reworked and understood in the present, help reshape one's understanding of the past and possibly even one's remembered experiences. In this sense, it is possible, so to speak, to reshape memories and thereby restructure personality.

In general, this process has been understood to involve at least two individuals. We believe, consistent with self-psychology, that under certain circumstances a single individual, having internalized the function of a significant other into his or her personality makeup, can and does reshape his or her own perceptions of the present and the past (Kohut, 1977; Basch, 1981). This achievement of personality restructuring epitomizes the therapeutic process and represents its crowning step: we have called it self-discovery.

This principle, the bidirectionality of effects, was at work with the Jordan family. By giving birth to Bobby, Mrs. Jordan had restored her feeling of femininity to herself, in part. She, too, now owned a male love object, just as her mother had (her brother). By letting Bobby play with her breasts, she gratified her need for being valued by someone she loved. (Bobby represented to her what her brother represented to her mother.) When Mrs. Jordan told her husband that she needed to be looked at, admired, and touched, she showed that she was finally able to repudiate the emptiness her mother had helped to create; she could now intercede on her own behalf, ask to be valued as a sexual woman by an appropriate object—her husband and not Bobby. Moreover, with her newly found capacity to experience with her husband and Bobby their own pain when they felt rejected, hurt, and depreciated, Mrs. Jordan was showing that she had come to value them too. In the process, she came full-circle back upon herself. Truly caring for others, she bestowed upon herself the capacity for self-love and self-care. A changed present had produced a changed past.

A similar process was noted with Mr. Jordan when he gently and lovingly set limits on Bobby without threatening to destroy him in the process. At that point, he saw the tension drain away from Bobby's shoulders and how easily the boy was then able to reimmerse himself in play. In behaving toward Bobby much differently than his own father or brother had toward him when he was a child, Mr. Jordan restored to himself a certain nonthreatening kindness which should have been part of his growing up experience but apparently was not. He had come to divest himself somehow of the autocratic, threatening, and punitive attitudes absorbed at the hands of his father and brother. In an act of love for his son Bobby, Mr. Jordan had also undone the early hurt inflicted on him. He became, as it were, his own father in the past and in the process had acquired a new parental image.

What accounted for the change in Bobby? With change occurring in his environment, Bobby's expectations based on the past were no longer fulfilled. He had to learn to perceive new contingencies in his environment. For his parents, he was no longer needed as buffer or bridge. His vigilance was no longer adaptive, and his roaming was now truly without purpose. For Bobby, the new task was to unlearn the past and learn about the present.

Unlike his mother and father, he was not called upon to forge new parental images for himself. This task would be met by his real parents in the real present.

To summarize, the structuring function of the psychic apparatus of the child between the ages of birth to three lies as much in the hands of the parents as it rests in the organizing capacities of the child. This view is based on much solid empirical research and new developments in interpersonal theory. To paraphrase Sanders (1975): The organization of behavior at the psychological level is not the property of the individual, rather it is the property of the more inclusive system of which the individual is a part.

The aim of this paper has been to illustrate from beginning to end, from assessment through treatment, how this personal and interpersonal theory and its various sub-principles illuminate clinical experience.

Outcome Evaluation and Last Contact

When the Jordan family completed treatment seventeen months after their initial evaluation in our program, reassessment revealed a newly cohesive unit whose members were much less stressed and significantly more satisfied with themselves and their relationships.

The outcome evaluation consisted of three parts: developmental testing for Bobby; a series of videotaped sequences of parent–child and family–child interaction; and a questionnaire designed to assess the parents' perceptions of our program and its effect on Bobby, on themselves as individuals, and on family relationships as a whole. Ratings on the Infant–Family Assessment Profile (see Table 7.1) are based on the scoring of the therapist and three other PIDS clinicians.

As can be seen in Table 7.1, gains were made across many areas of functioning by all three members of this moderately disturbed family. (For the sake of brevity, we confine ourselves once again to summarizing our clinical impressions without documenting in full the clinical observations that led to the rating of each and every aspect of functioning.)

THE INDIVIDUALS IN THE FAMILY

On individual lines, both Bobby and his parents had improved in the areas of affect and social relatedness. In the area of attachment, Bobby seemed more secure and less vigilant.

At age two years, eight months, Bobby was an energetic, engaging, and highly verbal little boy, still strikingly handsome and well coordinated. During testing with the Stanford–Binet, he was generally pleasant, enjoyed his accomplishments, and was responsive to and cooperative with the examiner. At times he had some difficulty sitting still and staying focused on a single task, but his unfocused roaming and hypervigilance had ceased. Bobby's IQ was 103 (CA = 2-8, MA = 3.2). While his best performance was on tasks of visual–motor coordination, all the items at his age level were completed.

Mrs. Jordan was seen now as less depressed and as having a greater sense of self-worth (including accepting herself as a loved and loving woman). Mr. Jordan's dysphoric feelings and his serious problems with dependency, self-esteem, and competence as a man had also been somewhat alleviated.

DSM-III diagnoses on all axes had changed for the better for all three members of the Jordan family (Spitzer, 1987).

RELATIONSHIPS WITHIN THE FAMILY

Mother and Bobby. Mrs. Jordan's presentation on outcome was strikingly different from her appearance and demeanor during the first evaluation. With her hair pinned off her face and dressed in a V-neck shirt and shorts, she seemed much more womanly and comfortable than before with both her sexuality and the maternal role. She moved with less restriction and more resolutely. Equally definite was her expectation that she and her son could enjoy themselves together at play.

Together with greater mutuality and a better dyadic fit, interaction between mother and child had improved specifically in the areas of reciprocal exchange, focalization, and recognition. When Bobby expressed interest in a wolf puppet during one of the final evaluation sessions, for instance, Mrs. Jordan had immersed herself in the game energetically and teasingly pretended to have the wolf "eat Bobby up." When her son ran away to hide under the table, she immediately tuned into the anxiety she had stirred up. "You don't want me to eat you up," she said and diverted the play to another, safer theme.

Mrs. Jordan's early unsuccessful attempts to make physical contact with Bobby using the wolf puppet did not discourage her from enjoying physical closeness with her son later. Both mother and child experienced great pleasure tickling each other (at Mrs. Jordan's initiative) and laughing together. As they continued playing, Mrs. Jordan was impressively flexible with Bobby. She affirmed, for example, that something he had found upsetting could be done later and also helped him express displeasure verbally rather than by acting out.

Mrs. Jordan handled her separation from Bobby sensitively and with forethought. She not only explained to Bobby that she would be gone briefly ("to the bathroom") and would return, but also attempted to set him working at a puzzle to occupy himself during her absence. It was a good separation. Bobby became upset, nonetheless, followed his mother out of the room, and insisted that, like his mother, he too had to use the bathroom.

Father and Bobby. Spontaneous and fun, Bobby's play with his father was marked by lots of laughter, teasing, and tickling. For the most part, the two boxed and tumbled, moving with little inhibition and much enjoyment. Mr. Jordan, who appeared relaxed and confident, interacted with his son in a way that was clearly familiar and pleasurable. The relationship between the two had clearly gained along the dimensions of self-assertiveness and recognition, as well.

As a teacher to his son, Mr. Jordan successfully captured Bobby's interest and both encouraged and challenged him. He also took sensitive advantage of a moment when the two were reading a book about babies to talk with Bobby (in anticipation of that upcoming event) about a new baby joining the family.

In contrast to his quick exit from the room in the separation sequence videotaped seventeen months before, Mr. Jordan explained to Bobby this time that he had to go briefly but would return. He also sat with him for a few moments to reflect his fears and reassure him that he would not be abandoned for good. Bobby protested his father's departure and clearly expressed his desire to join him ("I want to go too."). After a few moments of distressed screaming, Bobby began working at the doorknob and persevered until he had successfully opened the door and could leave the room. Upon his return, Mr. Jordan helped Bobby put into words his anxiety over the separation and reinforced the notion that they could think of each other when apart. "You didn't want me to be gone," Mr. Jordan said as he comforted his son. "I missed you."

Bobby and Family. When the whole family got together to play and have a snack, the tone was one of excited anticipation. There was a sense of newfound pleasure at being together, without the tensions and disappointments that had marred their interactions before. Mr. and Mrs. Jordan now had greater self-assurance in imparting their expectations to the child (see Table 7.1, "Internal Representation of the Parent"). Perhaps bolstered by the presence of the two parents at ease with one another, Bobby once again gravitated to the wolf puppet, but this time felt braver and more comfortable. "I'm going to get Mommy's nose," Bobby said. "I'm going to get Mommy's nose, too!," said his father as he gave her nose a tweak. Mrs. Jordan laughed with pleasure. The mock-teasing continued with her encouragement.

We saw Bobby as testing his muscles, showing his love, and providing evident signs of anxiety, as, still unable to tolerate the brief separation, he played at moving away from his parents.

Marital Relationship. The greatest change had occurred without a doubt in the Jordan's marital relations. They were now attuned to each other and their respective needs and wishes, as well as to their anxieties. They enjoyed each other's company and no longer needed to use Bobby as a go-between to diffuse their tensions and fuel their love. Availability to one another, communication, carrying out daily routines, setting family goals, and establishing alliances all had improved markedly.

Our overall impression was that both parents had begun to enjoy each other once again and were sharing mutual pride and pleasure in their little boy.

SOCIAL SUPPORTS AND LIVING CONDITIONS

The Jordans had begun treatment already relatively well situated with social supports and environmental conditions. One might not have expected much positive change in those areas, but here too there was improvement. Mrs. Jordan reported increased intimacy with her friends and Mr. Jordan had fewer problems with authority figures at work. Extended family relationships remained distant.

Now accustomed to bringing in two salaries, they no longer experienced Mrs. Jordan's employment as a sign of being in financial straits. Their home environment, while physically unchanged, and still as well equipped as before, was now a more emotionally pleasant and enjoyable place.

The Outcome Interview. In response to direct inquiry about the family's progress, both parents agreed that their presenting complaint—Bobby's insufficient affection and his rejection of their overtures—had ceased to be a problem almost from the beginning. Mr. Jordan noted that his son now expressed affection "readily and freely both verbally and physically." Mrs. Jordan pointed out that Bobby expressed anger too—an important observation for a woman who, at intake, had been so constricted and inhibited in her own expression of feelings.

Mr. Jordan had some minor concerns about Bobby's "disrespect for his toys," but qualified his statement with a reminder to himself out loud that his son was "still learning." Mrs. Jordan was pleased to report that Bobby had begun to carry his own pillow around the house instead of one of theirs. She seemed to be showing her pleasure over Bobby's budding autonomy while still acknowledging his appropriate need for dependence and support.

The most valuable part of infant–family therapy for Bobby, according to Mr. Jordan, was that "Bobby could see we had feelings we had to deal with. As a result of us dealing with our feelings, he could do the same." In this statement, Mr. Jordan revealed his awareness of the impact on Bobby of the past marital conflict and his sense of being an important role model for the boy.

Mrs. Jordan, on the other hand, felt that the most important effect of infant–family therapy on Bobby was "our being able to communicate to each other both good and bad feelings—our being able to observe and reflect his feelings, like saying, 'You're mad!' " Her emphasis on the emotion of anger and her increasing comfort in expressing it were of great significance to Mrs. Jordan. She felt she had been helped personally by our program, particularly "because (she) needed to get rid of so much anger." She went on to say that she now knew that if "I yell or say something that might hurt (my husband's) feelings, he won't hate me." The great fear of rejection that had led to her previously tough and unapproachable stance was clearly diminishing.

Mr. Jordan felt that their marital problems had been "resolved for the most part. There are still some difficulties," he continued, "but we can *discuss* them. A cloud seems to have been lifted." The cloud to which he was referring was apparently his own self-doubt. It was giving way to a newly acquired ability for self-assertion and for taking risks he had previously thought impossible.

Both Mr. and Mrs. Jordan felt that all three family members were "very much better" as a result of their participation in our program. They gave themselves the highest possible rating for progress (a "1" on a 6-point scale). They ended their contact with us describing talking together on the front steps of a summer's evening, hugging before bed, and making plans for the arrival of their new baby. They sounded genuinely content.

References

American Psychiatric Association (1980), *The Diagnostic and Statistical Manual of Mental Disorders* (DSM-III), 3rd ed. Washington, DC: American Psychiatric Press.

Basch, M. F. (1981), Psychoanalytic interpretation and cognitive transformation. *Internat. J. Psycho-Anal.*, 62:151–175.

——— (1983), Empathic understanding: A review of the concept and some theoretical considerations. *Internat. J. Psycho-Anal.*, 64:101–127.

Beckwith, L. (1972), Relationships between infants' social behavior and their mothers' behavior. *Child Develop.*, 43:397–411.

Bell, R. W. (1968), A reinterpretation of the direction of effects in studies of socialization. *Psycholog. Rev.*, 74:81–95.

Belsky, J. (1979), The interrelation of parental and spousal behavior during infancy in traditional nuclear families: An exploratory analysis. *J. Marr. & Fam.*, 41:62–68.

——— (1981), Early human experience: A family perspective. *Development. Psychol.*, 17:3–23.

Benedek, T. (1959), Parenthood as a developmental phase. *J. Amer. Psychoanal. Assn.*, 78:389–417.

——— (1970), Parenthood during the life cycle. In: *Parenthood: Its Psychology and Psychopathology*, ed. E. J. Anthony & T. Benedek. Boston: Little, Brown.

Bertalanffy, L. von (1968), *General Systems Theory: Foundations, Development Applications*. New York: George Braziller.

Brazelton, T. B., Koslowski, B., & Main, M. (1974), The origins of reciprocity in the mother-infant interaction. In: *The Effect of the Infant on the Caregiver*, Vol. 1, ed. M. Lewis & L. Rosenblum. New York: John Wiley.

Buie, D. H. (1981), Empathy: Its nature and limitations. *J. Amer. Psychoanal. Assn.*, 29:281–308.

Clark-Stewart, K. A. (1973), Interactions between mothers and their young children: Characteristics and consequences. *Monographs of the Society for Research in Child Development*, 38 (Serial No. 153).

Emde, R. (1981), Emotional availability: A reciprocal reward system for infants and parents with implications for prevention of psychosocial disorders. In: *Parent–Infant Relationships*, ed. P. Taylor. New York: Grune & Stratton.

Fraiberg, S. (1980), *Clinical Studies in Infant Mental Health: The First Year of Life*. New York: Basic Books.

——— Adelson, E., & Shapiro, V. (1975), Ghosts in the nursery. *J. Amer. Acad. Child Psychiat.*, 14:387–421.

Greenspan, S. (1981), *Psychopathology and Adaptation in Infancy and Early Childhood: Principles of Clinical Diagnosis and Preventive Intervention*. New York: International Universities Press.

Jaffe, D. S. (1968), The mechanism of projection: Its dual role in object relations. *Internat. J. Psycho-Anal.*, 49:662–677.

Jessner, L., Weigert, E., & Foy, J. L. (1970), The development of parental attitudes during pregnancy. In: *Parenthood: Its Psychology and Psychopathology*, ed. E. J. Anthony & T. Benedek. Boston: Little, Brown.

Klein, M. (1946), Notes on some schizoid mechanisms. *Internat. J. Psycho-Anal.*, 27:99–110.

Kohut, H. (1959), Introspection, empathy, and psychoanalysis. *J. Amer. Psychoanal. Assn.*, 7:459–483.

——— (1977), *The Restoration of the Self*. New York: International Universities Press.

Lerner, R. M., & Spanier, G. B. (1978), A dynamic interactional view of child and family development. In: *Child Influences on Marital*

and *Family Interactions: A Life-Span Perspective*, ed. R. M. Lerner &
G. B. Spanier. New York: Academic Press.

Lidz, T. (1976), *The Person: His and Her Development Throughout the Life-Cycle*, rev. ed. New York: Basic Books.

Roth, C. H., Levin, D. S., Morrison, M., & Leventhal, B. L., Interventions for infants and their families: A systems approach. (Submitted.)

Sameroff, A. J. (1982), Development and the dialectic: The need for a systems approach. In: *The Concept of Development*, Vol. 15, ed. W. A. Collins. Minnesota Symposia on Child Development. Minneapolis, MN: University of Minnesota Press.

——— Chandler, M. J. (1975), Reproductive risks and the continuum of caretaking casualty. In: *Review of Child Development*, Vol. 4, ed. F. D. Horowitz. Chicago: University of Chicago Press.

——— Harris, A. E. (1979), Dialectical approaches to early thought and language. In: *Psychological Development From Infancy: Image to Intention*, ed. M. H. Bornstein & W. Kessen. Hillsdale, NJ: Lawrence Erlbaum Associates.

Sander, K. (1983), Polarity, paradox and organizing process in development. In: *Frontiers of Infant Psychiatry*, ed. J. D. Call, E. Galenson, & R. L. Tyson. New York: Basic Books.

Sanders, L. W. (1975), Infant and caretaking environment: Investigation and conceptualization of adaptive behavior in a system of increasing complexity. In: *Exploration in Child Psychiatry*, ed. E. J. Anthony. New York: Plenum Press.

Schafer, R. (1978), *Language and Insight*. New Haven, CT: Yale University Press.

——— (1982), The relevance of the "here and now" transference interpretation to the reconstruction of early development. *Internat. J. Psycho-Anal.*, 63:77–82.

Spence, D. P. (1982), Narrative truth and theoretical truth. *Psychoanal. Quart.*, 51:43–68.

Spitzer, R. L. (1981), *DSM III Casebook*. Washington, DC: American Psychiatric Press.

——— (1987), *Diagnostic and Statistical Manual of Mental Disorders (DSM III-R)*. Washington, DC: American Psychiatric Association, Press.

Sroufe, L. A. (1979), The coherence of individual development: Early care, attachment and subsequent developmental issues. *Amer. Psycholog.*, 34:834–841.

Stern, D. (1977), *The First Relationship*. Cambridge, MA: Harvard University Press.

——— (1983), The early development of schemas of self, other, and "self with other." In: *Reflections and Self Psychology*, ed. J. D. Lichtenberg & S. Kaplan. New York: International Universities Press.

Winnicott, D. W. (1958), *Through Pediatrics to Psychoanalysis*. London: Hogarth Press.

Zinner, J., & Shapiro, R. (1972), Projective identification as a mode of perception and behaviour in families of adolescents. *Internat. J. Psycho-Anal.*, 53:523–530.

Name Index

303

Subject Index